Objective Tests for Nurses
Book Two

Other books in the series contain questions on anatomy and physiology, and nursing care of medical and surgical conditions related to the following body systems:

Book One: The structure of the body

Forthcoming titles

Book Three: The circulatory system and the respiratory system

Book Four: The digestive system and the urinary system

Book Five: The nervous system and the special senses

Book Six: The endocrine system and the female reproductive system

Objective Tests for Nurses
Book Two

The skeletal system and the muscular system

Janet T. E. Riddle

RGN RFN ONC RNT (Edin)
Formerly senior tutor, College of Nursing and Midwifery,
Greater Glasgow Health Board, Western District

The late **Joan Dinner**

SRN RCNT
Formerly assessor to the General Nursing Council for England and Wales. Approved lecturer to the British Red Cross Society. Clinical teacher, Royal Hampshire County Hospital, Winchester. Formerly ward sister, Victoria Hospital, Winchester

Foreword by Margaret W. Thomson

RGN RSCN RNT SCM
Registrar, General Nursing Council for Scotland

CHURCHILL LIVINGSTONE
EDINBURGH LONDON MELBOURNE AND NEW YORK 1981

CHURCHILL LIVINGSTONE
Medical Division of Longman Group Limited

Distributed in the United States of America by
Churchill Livingstone Inc., 19 West 44th Street,
New York, N.Y. 10036, and by associated
companies, branches and representatives throughout
the world.

© Longman Group Limited, 1981

All rights reserved. No part of this publication may
be reproduced, stored in a retrieval system, or
transmitted in any form or by any means, electronic,
mechanical, photocopying, recording or otherwise,
without the prior permission of the publishers
(Churchill Livingstone, Robert Stevenson House,
1–3 Baxter's Place, Leith Walk, Edinburgh, EH1 3AF).

First published 1981

ISBN 0 443 01740 9

British Library Cataloguing in Publication Data

Riddle, Janet Thomson Elliot
  Objective tests for nurses.
  Book 2: The skeletal system and the muscular
  system
  1. Nursing—Problems, exercises, etc.
  I. Title
  II. Dinner, Joan
  610.73'076 RT55 80-40910

Printed in Singapore by
Singapore Offset Printing Pte Ltd

Foreword

The process of nursing has led nurses and nurse educators to be much more aware of the need to be objective in their approach to solving problems relating to nursing care given to patients. Since the first written examination for nurses, leading to Registration with the General Nursing Council for Scotland, was held in 1925, the Council has endeavoured to construct a reliable means of ascertaining that candidates have reached a level of proficiency which will enable them to practise safely as Registered or Enrolled nurses.

The present system of examination consists of a written paper and a continuous assessment of proficiency in practice in the clinical areas: the former to test knowledge of facts and the understanding of the application of these facts to nursing practice, the latter to assess skills and attitudes which can more properly be assessed in a clinical setting.

The Council set up the Panel of Examiners which has given consideration to the format of the questions in the written paper and to the difficulties of their construction and marking relative to the various types.

The Council welcomed Churchill Livingstone's approach to assist in the compilation of a book which would be of interest to learners and assist them in their preparation to become Registered or Enrolled nurses. In order to encourage nurse teachers to participate in the compilation of the book, a workshop was sponsored by Churchill Livingstone under the auspices of the Department of Psychology at Moray House College of Education.

Although the General Nursing Council for Scotland has not so far included multiple choice questions in the final paper, the benefit to be gained from utilising this book as a learning aid is to be commended. I trust that it will assist the learners to develop a questioning attitude and indeed provide some of the answers in order that they may become competent practitioners of nursing.

Margaret W. Thomson

About the series

Foreword

This series of books was devised in response to the ever-increasing demand for books which would give the nurse learner practice in answering objective tests. Each book in the series consists of questions on two body systems. Within each system the questions are split into (1) those on anatomy and physiology and (2) those on case histories based on common disorders relating to each system.

However, the authors and publishers felt that in order to be really useful the books should be more than just a collection of questions and answers. We wanted the reader to be able to find out *why* one answer was considered right and another wrong and to understand the implications involved. For this reason the nursing care questions have been based on case histories and full explanatory answers are given in these sections.

Since we regarded the books as aids to learning and revision rather than as 'crammers' for examinations, we have not confined ourselves to the use of multiple choice questions only. Instead a variety of objective tests has been used and again it is hoped that this will make the books more interesting and useful to the reader.

The questions have been tested on different groups of nurse learners and all have been found to be appropriate. No attempt has been made to grade the questions; they have been written for the nurse learner who has completed the first eighteen months of training. All the results have been evaluated by computer and subsequently analysed and any questions of doubtful ambiguity have been omitted.

Finally we felt it to be most important that the page layout used should provide space for the reader to make individual notes against the questions. For this reason we have used a page size considerably larger than is usual in books of this type.

We would emphasise that the book should be used in conjunction with other texts. A pre-knowledge of anatomy and physiology has been assumed and for further reference the reader is referred to the books in the short bibliography all of which are published by Churchill Livingstone.

Bibliography

Bloom: *Toohey's Medicine for Nurses*
Moroney: *Surgery for Nurses*
Riddle: *Anatomy and Physiology Applied to Nursing*
Ross and Wilson: *Foundations of Anatomy and Physiology*
Chilman and Thomas: *Understanding Nursing Care*

Preface

The authors of this book have experimented for a number of years with different types of objective test questions. Now that this form of examination paper is becoming more popular there is a need to produce questions for student and pupil nurses to use for practice and revision. Most of the available books are geared to the needs of the medical students or are American publications couched in unfamiliar terminology.

Although the main part of the book deals with nursing some anatomy and physiology questions are included. These are very basic and are aimed at testing the student's previous knowledge of the subjects. The questions should be studied with a textbook on hand for reference, revision and further study.

In the nursing care studies the author has attempted to cover many aspects of nursing care and to form questions which test knowledge of facts, principles, understanding and evaluation. She has explained, in some detail, why she has selected the correct answer. The student may not always agree with her, but it should be remembered that this book is not an examination and it is hoped that it will stimulate study and discussion.

We would like to express our gratitude to Mary Emmerson Law of Churchill Livingstone who has not only edited the book and encouraged the authors but has also spent a considerable amount of time having the questions tested and evaluated. Without her enthusiasm this book may never have been written.

We wish to thank the following people: Miss M. Thomson of the General Nursing Council for Scotland and Miss Win Logan of the International Council of Nurses (formerly of the Scottish Home and Health Department) for their interest; the nurses who took the tests and the tutors who administered them; Mr Coulthard of Moray House College of Education and the college computer operators for their help in evaluating the test results; Miss J. Ross and Dr K. Wilson for allowing us to use some of their illustrations and lastly our friends who helped and encouraged—especially Miss J. Barnwell, Mrs M. Dickson and Miss K. Nicoll.

Numerous people have given expert advice and Miss Dinner would particularly like to thank Mrs C. Dobson, Librarian, and all the staff of the Post-Graduate Library at the Royal Hampshire County Hospital, Winchester, who have far exceeded the call of duty with their enthusiasm and willingness to help.

January 1980
Janet T. E. Riddle
Joan Dinner

Postscript

Since the work on the writing and compilation of this book was completed I have to record the sudden and unexpected death of my co-author, Joan Dinner. Her enthusiasm for the series played an important part in its development and it is sad to note that she died before any of the books which she had helped to write could be published.

March 1980
Janet T. E. Riddle

Contents

Anatomy and physiology of bones, joints and muscles

Multiple choice questions

The following questions (1–20) are all of the multiple choice type. Read the questions, and from the possible answers select the ONE which you think is correct. You may indicate your answer by writing the appropriate letter in the right hand margin. The answers to these questions may be found on page 19.

1. A rough projection of bone is called:
   A. An articulation
   B. A foramen
   C. A suture
   D. A tubercle.

   1.

2. A depression in a bone is called a:
   A. Foramen
   B. Fossa
   C. Meatus
   D. Sinus.

   2.

3. A small flat articulating surface on a bone is called a:
   A. Facet
   B. Fissure
   C. Process
   D. Septum.

   3.

4. The only movable bone of the skull is the:
   A. Lachrymal
   B. Mandible
   C. Maxillary
   D. Temporal.

   4.

5. The bone which forms the supraorbital ridges of the skull is the:
   A. Frontal
   B. Occipital
   C. Parietal
   D. Temporal.

   5.

6. Which one of the following statements is true of the curves of the spine?
   A. The cervical curve is concave forwards
   B. The lumbar curve appears at three months
   C. The thoracic curve is a primary curve
   D. The sacral curve is a secondary curve.

   6.

7. The ribs are:
   A. Flat bones
   B. Irregular bones
   C. Long bones
   D. Short bones.

7.

8. The olecranon is part of the:
   A. Humerus
   B. Radius
   C. Scapula
   D. Ulna.

8.

9. The head of the ulna is on the:
   A. Lateral side of the elbow
   B. Lateral side of the wrist
   C. Medial side of the elbow
   D. Medial side of the wrist.

9.

10. Which of the following joints are fibrous?
    A. The radioulnar joints
    B. The intervertebral joints
    C. The joints of the toes
    D. The sutures of the skull.

10.

11. Which one of the following statements is true?
    A. A cartilaginous joint gives no movement
    B. A fibrous joint has a capsule
    C. A fixed joint has a pad of cartilage
    D. A freely movable joint has a synovial lining.

11.

12. One of the movements possible at the elbow joint is:
    A. Abduction
    B. Circumduction
    C. Extension
    D. Rotation.

12.

13. The radioulnar joints are:
    A. Condyloid
    B. Gliding
    C. Hinge
    D. Pivot.

13.

14. At the wrist joint all the following movements are possible except one. Which one?
    A. Abduction
    B. Adduction
    C. Flexion
    D. Rotation.

14.

15. One of the waste products of muscle contraction is:
    A. Carbon monoxide
    B. Glucose
    C. Oxygen
    D. Water.

15.

16. The deltoid is a:
    A. A long straight muscle
    B. Rectangular muscle
    C. Round muscle
    D. Triangular muscle.

16.

17. The biceps muscle:
    A. Extends the elbow
    B. Flexes the wrist
    C. Extends the shoulder
    D. Supinates the forearm.

17.

18. The anterior abdominal muscles have many functions. Which of the following is incorrect?
    A. They extend the spine
    B. They contract in coughing
    C. They contract in defaecation
    D. They assist in respiration.

18.

19. The gluteal muscles:
    A. Cover the sciatic nerve
    B. Are four in number
    C. Are supplied by the femoral nerve
    D. Lie in front of the hip joint.

19

20. The quadriceps muscle:
    A. Extends the hip
    B. Extends the knee
    C. Abducts the hip
    D. Flexes the knee.

20.

Matching item questions

The following questions (21–57) are all of the matching item type. They consist of two lists. On the left is a list of lettered items (A, B, C etc.). On the right is a list of numbered items. Study the two lists and for each item in the numbered list select the appropriate item from the lettered list. You may indicate your answer by writing the appropriate letter in the right hand margin.

Note. There are more items in the lettered list than in the numbered lists and you will therefore not use all the items in the lettered list.

21–23. From the list on the left select the word whose meaning most closely approximates to the word in the list on the right.

A. Above	21. Medial	21.
B. Below		
C. Behind	22. Posterior	22.
D. In front		
E. In the centre.	23. Superior.	23.

24–26. From the list on the left select the word which is used to classify each bone on the right.

A. Flat	24. Patella	24.
B. Irregular		
C. Long	25. Radius	25.
D. Sesamoid		
E. Short.	26. Vertebra.	26.

27–29. From the list on the left select the function which is applicable to each structure on the right.

A. Contains yellow bone marrow	27. Hyaline cartilage	27.
B. Forms a passage for the blood supply to compact bone tissue		
C. Contributes to the formation of joints	28. Periosteum	28.
D. Contains developing red blood cells		
E. Strengthens the bone.	29. Red bone marrow.	29.

30–32. From the list on the right select the bones of the skull which are joined by the sutures listed on the left.

A. Frontal and parietal	30. Coronal	30.
B. Right parietal and left parietal		
C. Occipital and parietal	31. Lambdoidal	31.
D. Temporal and sphenoid		
E. Temporal and parietal.	32. Sagittal.	32.

33–35. From the list on the left select the structures which form the boundaries of the thorax.

A. Diaphragm   33. Anterior   33.
B. Ribs
C. Sternum   34. Inferior   34.
D. Trachea
E. Vertebrae.   35. Posterior.   35.

36–38. From the list on the left select an organ situated in each cavity on the right.

A. Larynx   36. Abdomen   36.
B. Lungs
C. Spleen   37. Pelvis   37.
D. Testes
E. Uterus   38. Thorax.   38.

39–41. From the list on the left select a part of each bone on the right.

A. Capitellum   39. Humerus   39.
B. Coracoid process
C. Costal groove   40. Rib   40.
D. Olecranon process
E. Xiphoid process.   41. Sternum.   41.

42–44. From the list on the left select a part of each bone on the right.

A. Anterior crest   42. Femur   42.
B. Intertrochanteric ridge
C. Lateral malleolus   43. Innominate bone   43.
D. Obturator foramen
E. Superior articulating process.   44. Tibia.   44.

45–47. From the list on the left select a joint belonging to each type of articulation on the right.

A. The ankle joint   45. Ball and socket   45.
B. The hip joint
C. The intervertebral joints   46. Condyloid   46.
D. The radioulnar joints
E. The wrist joint.   47. Hinge.   47.

48–51. From the list on the left select a movement which can be described by each word on the right.

A. Arm moves towards the trunk   48. Abduction   48.
B. Foot turned in
C. Knee bent   49. Flexion   49.
D. Palm turned up   50. Inversion   50.
E. Thigh moves away from the
    midline.   51. Supination.   51.

52–54. From the list on the left select a movement which can be produced by
each muscle on the right.
A. Abduction of the shoulder   52. Deltoid   52.
B. Extension of the elbow
C. Extension of the hip   53. Gluteals   33.
D. Flexion of the knee.   54. Hamstrings   54.

55–57. From the list on the left select a movement which can be produced by
each muscle on the right.
A. Flexion of the elbow   55. Trapezius   55.
B. Plantar flexion of the ankle
C. Raising the shoulder girdle   56. Triceps   56.
D. Extension of the elbow   57. Biceps.   57.

Matching item questions using a diagram

The following questions (58–119) all consist of a diagram with numbered parts. With each diagram there is a list of named parts (A, B, C etc.). Look at the diagram and for each numbered structure select a name from the list of parts. You may indicate your answer by writing the appropriate letter in the right hand margin.

Note. There are more lettered items than numbers on the diagram so you will not use all the names in the lists.

58–60. A section through a long bone
    A. Compact bone tissue
    B. Hyaline cartilage
    C. Medullary canal
    D. Periosteum
    E. Red bone marrow.

58.

59.

60.

61–63. A growing bone
    A. Diaphysis
    B. Epiphysis
    C. Epiphyseal cartilage
    D. Primary centre of ossification
    E. Secondary centre of ossification.

61.

62.

63.

64–66. The vault of an infant's skull
    A. Anterior fontanelle
    B. Frontal bone
    C. Occipital bone
    D. Parietal bone
    E. Suture.

64.

65.

66.

ANTERIOR

POSTERIOR

67–69. A typical cervical vertebra
    A. The body
    B. The neural arch
    C. The neural canal
    D. The spinous process.

67.

68.

69.

70–72. Longitudinal section through the spine
    A. Anterior longitudinal ligament
    B. Interspinous ligament
    C. Intervertebral disc
    D. Posterior longitudinal ligament
    E. Supraspinous ligament.

70.

71.

72.

73–75. The scapula
    A. Acromion process
    B. Coracoid process
    C. Glenoid cavity
    D. Infraspinous fossa
    E. Inferior angle.

73.

74.

75.

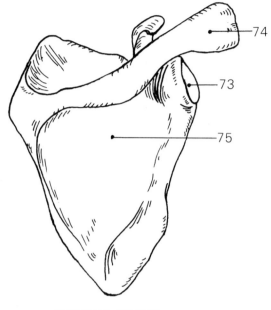

POSTERIOR SURFACE

76–78. The humerus
    A. The articulating surface for the scapula
    B. The articulating surface for the ulna
    C. The greater tuberosity
    D. The articulating surface for the radius
    E. The medial epicondyle.

76.

77.

78.

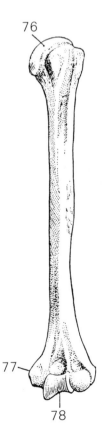

79–81. The radius and ulna
    A. Coronoid process
    B. Head of radius
    C. Head of ulna
    D. Olecranon
    E. Radial tubercle.

79.

80.

81.

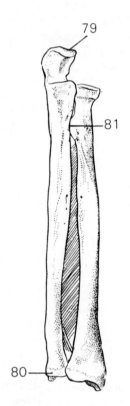

82–84. The innominate bone
    A. The acetabulum
    B. The ischial tuberosity
    C. The posterior superior iliac spine
    D. The pubic tubercle
    E. The sciatic notch.

82.

83.

84.

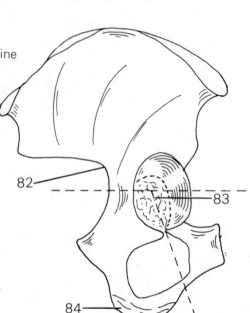

85–87. The femur
    A. The greater trochanter
    B. The linea aspera
    C. The medial condyle
    D. The patellar surface
    E. The popliteal surface.

85.

86.

87.

88–90. The tibia and fibula
    A. Interosseous membrane
    B. Lateral malleolus
    C. Medial condyle
    D. Tibial crest
    E. Tibial tubercle.

88.

89.

90.

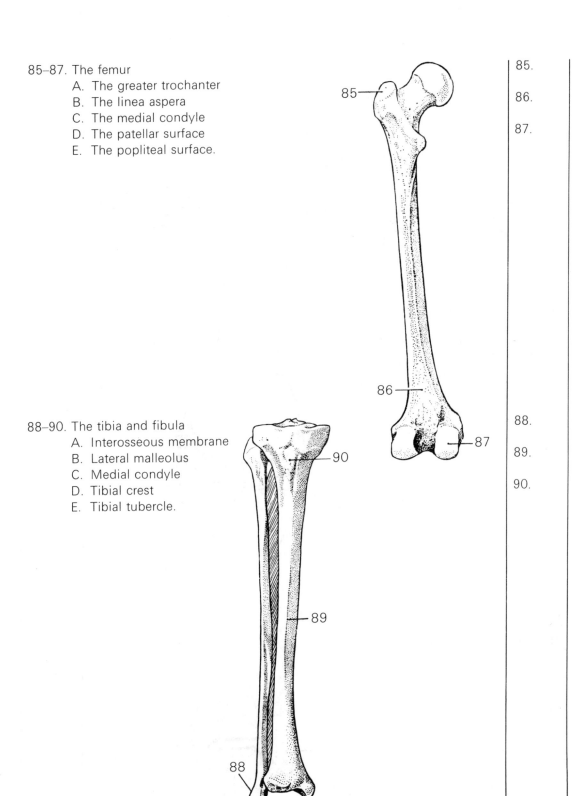

91–93. Bones of the foot
    A. Calcaneus
    B. Cuboid
    C. Metatarsals
    D. Phalanges
    E. Talus.

91.

92.

93.

94–97. A synovial joint
    A. Capsule
    B. Extracapsular ligament
    C. Hyaline cartilage
    D. Synovial fluid
    E. Synovial membrane.

94.

95.

96.

97.

98–100. The ankle joint
    A. Calcaneus
    B. Lateral malleolus
    C. Medial malleolus
    D. Talus.

98.

99.

100.

101–104. Muscles of the trunk and limbs
     A. Biceps
     B. Deltoid
     C. Gluteals
     D. Hamstrings
     E. Anterior abdominal wall.

101.

102.

103.

104.

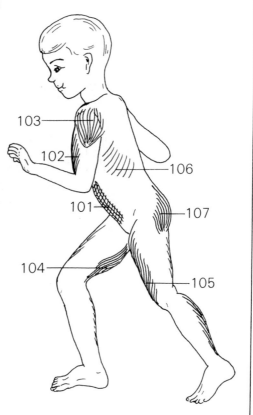

105–107. Muscles of the trunk and limbs (see diagram above)
     A. Quadriceps
     B. Trapezius
     C. Triceps
     D. Intercostals
     E. Gluteals.

105.

106.

107.

108–110. The diaphragm
    A. Aorta
    B. 10th rib
    C. 11th rib
    D. Sternum.

108.

109.

110.

111–113. The diaphragm (see diagram above)
    A. Lumbar vertebra
    B. Oesophagus
    C. Thoracic vertebra
    D. Vena cava.

111.

112.

113.

114–116. The pelvic floor
    A. Anus
    B. Levator ani muscles
    C. Perineum
    D. Peritoneum.

114.

115.

116.

117–119. The pelvic floor (see diagram above)
    A. Sacrum
    B. Symphysis pubis
    C. Urethra
    D. Vagina.

117.

118.

119.

True false questions

The following questions (120–179) consist of a number of statements, some of which are true and some of which are false. Consider each statement and decide whether you think it is true or false. You can indicate your answer by writing T for true or F for false in the right hand margin beside each statement.

120–123. In the skull:
    120. The ethmoid is one of the bones of the cranium   120.

    121. The foramen magnum is in the parietal bone   121.

    122. The optic foramena are in the sphenoid bone   122.

    123. The organ of hearing is situated in the temporal bone.   123.

124–127. Air sinuses are present in the following skull bones:
    124. Ethmoid   124.

    125. Maxillary   125.

    126. Occipital   126.

    127. Parietal.   127.

128–131. In the vertebral column there are:
    128. 7 cervical vertebrae   128.

    129. 12 lumbar vertebrae   129.

    130. 5 sacral vertebrae   130.

    131. 5 thoracic vertebrae.   131.

132–135. The sternum:
    132. Consists of three parts   132.

    133. Has attachments for all the ribs   133.

    134. Is a flat bone   134.

    135. Lies in front of the heart.   135.

136–139. The radius:

    136. Articulates with the humerus   136.

    137. Articulates with the head of the ulna   137.

    138. Articulates with the upper extremity of the ulna   138.

    139. Articulates with the medial two carpal bones.   139.

140–143. The female pelvis:

    140. Is smaller than the male pelvis   140.

    141. Has a cylindrical cavity   141.

    142. Has a narrow pubic arch   142.

    143. Has a more concave sacrum than the male pelvis.   143.

144–147. The parts which make up the innominate bone are:

    144. The ilium   144.

    145. The ischium   145.

    146. The pubis   146.

    147. The sacrum.   147.

148–151. The innominate bone:

    148. Is made up of three flat bones   148.

    149. The ilium contains the obturator foramen   149.

    150. The ischium takes the weight in the sitting position   150.

    151. The ilium is the origin of the gluteal muscles.   151.

152–155. One foot:

    152. Has 8 tarsal bones   152.

    153. Has 3 arches   153.

    154. Has 15 short bones forming the toes   154.

    155. Has 5 metatarsals.   155.

156–159. The movements possible at synovial joints are:
156. At a pivot joint—abduction

      156.

157. At a hinge joint—circumduction

      157.

158. At a condyloid joint—flexion

      158.

159. At a ball and socket joint—rotation.

      159.

160–163. The shoulder joint is:
160. A ball and socket joint

      160.

161. The joint between the head of the humerus and the acromion process

      161.

162. The joint between the head of the humerus and the glenoid cavity

      162.

163. A synovial joint.

      163.

164–167. In the hip joint:
164. The capsule is strengthened by ligaments

      164.

165. There is a depression in the head of the femur

      165.

166. The socket is deepened by a ring of fibrocartilage

      166.

167. The hyaline cartilage covers the whole of the acetabulum.

      167.

168–171. The knee joint:
168. Is a synovial gliding joint

      168.

169. Is extended when the leg is bent

      169.

170. Has two menisci

      170.

171. Is an articulation between three bones.

      171.

172–175. When a muscle contracts:
172. Glucose is broken down

      172.

173. Heat is given off

      173.

174. It uses up carbon dioxide

      174.

175. Water is a waste product.

      175.

176–179. The diaphragm:

    176. Is a sheet of voluntary muscle tissue   176.

    177. Relaxes during expiration   177.

    178. Contracts when the intercostal muscles relax   178.

    179. Rises when it contracts.   179.

Answers (Questions 1 to 179)

Multiple choice *(Page 1)*

1. D	6. C	11. D	16. D
2. B	7. A	12. C	17. D
3. A	8. D	13. D	18. A
4. B	9. D	14. D	19. A
5. A	10. D	15. D	20. B

Matching items *(Page 4)*

21. E	31. C	41. E	51. D
22. C	32. B	42. B	52. A
23. A	33. C	43. D	53. C
24. D	34. A	44. A	54. D
25. C	35. E	45. B	55. C
26. B	36. C	46. E	56. D
27. C	37. E	47. A	57. A
28. B	38. B	48. E	
29. D	39. A	49. C	
30. A	40. C	50. B	

Matching items using a diagram *(Page 7)*

58. D	74. A	90. E	106. D
59. B	75. D	91. E	107. E
60. C	76. A	92. C	108. A
61. B	77. E	93. A	109. D
62. A	78. B	94. B	110. C
63. C	79. D	95. A	111. B
64. A	80. C	96. E	112. A
65. E	81. E	97. C	113. D
66. C	82. E	98. C	114. B
67. A	83. A	99. B	115. A
68. C	84. B	100. D	116. C
69. D	85. A	101. E	117. D
70. C	86. E	102. A	118. C
71. B	87. C	103. B	119. B
72. E	88. B	104. D	
73. C	89. D	105. A	

True false *(Page 15)*

120. True	123. True	126. False	129. False
121. False	124. True	127. False	130. True
122. True	125. True	128. True	131. False

132. True	144. True	156. False	168. False
133. False	145. True	157. False	169. False
134. True	146. True	158. True	170. True
135. True	147. False	159. True	171. True
136. True	148. False	160. True	172. True
137. True	149. False	161. False	173. True
138. True	150. True	162. True	174. False
139. False	151. True	163. True	175. True
140. False	152. False	164. True	176. True
141. True	153. True	165. True	177. True
142. False	154. False	166. True	178. False
143. True	155. True	167. False	179. False

Congenital dislocation of the hip

The following questions (180–211) are based on the case history given below.

Mr and Mrs Lloyd had been married for two years, and owned a semi-detached house on the outskirts of a large city. They were both aged 24 years and eagerly awaited the birth of their first child. They were hoping for a baby girl, but their main concern was that the baby should be healthy whatever it's sex. At times they did feel rather anxious about this because Mrs Lloyd had had a congenital dislocation of the hip, and had spent much of her early life in hospital. She still walked with a slight limp.

On the 10th August 1978, Mrs Lloyd gave birth to a baby girl who weighed 3.5 kilogrammes. Both parents were delighted and named their baby Tracey.

True false questions

The following questions (180–187) consist of a number of statements, some of which are true and some of which are false. Consider each statement and decide whether you think it is true or false. You can indicate your answer by writing T for true or F for false in the right hand margin beside each statement.

180. The incidence of congenital dislocation of the hip is equally common among children of both sexes. | 180.

181. A woman who has had a congenital dislocation of the hip is unlikely to have children with this disability. | 181.

182. When congenital dislocation of the hip is diagnosed, there is frequently a history that the child was born in the breech position. | 182.

183. Women who have been treated for congenital dislocation of the hip in childhood must always have their children delivered by caesarean section. | 183.

184. Congenital dislocation of the hip is caused by the mother being exposed to the morbilli virus during the first 12 weeks of pregnancy. | 184.

185. Congenital dislocation of the hip is more commonly unilateral than bilateral. | 185.

186. There is a higher incidence of congenital dislocation of the hip in the British Isles than in any other part of the world. | 186.

187. It is rare for a diagnosis of congenital dislocation of the hip to be confirmed before the child reaches the age of 10 months. | 187.

When Tracey was 5 days old the doctor told Mr and Mrs Lloyd that he felt their daughter should be seen by an orthopaedic surgeon. In due course Tracey was examined and a diagnosis of bilateral congenital dislocation of the hips was made.

Mr and Mrs Lloyd were naturally very distressed, and the surgeon explained that although Tracey would need a long period of treatment it would be possible for her to be cared for at home for most of the time.

For the first year Tracey could remain at home and attend the hospital outpatient department at four-monthly intervals for review. She would need to wear 'double nappies' and lie in the prone position.

Multiple choice questions

The following questions (188–211) are based on the subsequent care of Tracey. They are all of the multiple choice type. Read the questions and from the possible answers select the ONE which you think is correct. You may indicate your answer by writing the appropriate number in the space provided or against the question number on your answer sheet.

188. Bearing in mind Tracey's age (5 days), which of the following would indicate a diagnosis of congenital dislocation of the hip?

    A positive sign of:
    A. Ortolani
    B. Kernig
    C. Babinski
    D. Trendelenburg.

188.

189. The purpose of nursing Tracey in double nappies is that the extra thickness will:
    A. Provide greater absorbency and so reduce the number of times her hips will need to be adducted for changing
    B. Increase the degree of abduction of the hips
    C. Provide greater support for the pelvic joints
    D. Prevent her from 'kicking'.

189.

190. Mrs Lloyd had been breast feeding her baby and was very anxious to
continue doing so, but was concerned that she might cause further injury to
Tracey's hip by holding her too closely against her body. In view of this,
which would be the best advice for the nurse to give to Mrs Lloyd?
    A. Worry about this will cause Mrs Lloyd's milk supply to decrease and
    therefore it would be better to bottle feed Tracey with an alternative to
    breast milk
    B. Bottle feed her with an alternative to breast milk while she is still young
    enough to adapt to the change of feeds, as it will be difficult to continue
    breast feeding when she needs to be admitted to hospital
    C. Leave Tracey in her cot at feed times and bottle feed her with expressed
    breast milk, as unnecessary handling of the baby should be avoided
    D. Continue to breast feed Tracey as she will benefit from the close contact
    with her mother.

190.

191. Tracey's birth weight was 3.5 kg. When she was 10 days old her weight
was still 3.5 kg. Which of the following statements provides the most
probable explanation for this?
    A. Her metabolic rate was higher than that of normal babies
    B. Babies normally lose a little weight in the first few days of life and
    regain it by the time they are 10 days old
    C. Babies with congenital dislocation of hip have a tendency to 'fail to
    thrive'
    D. Tracey needed extra nourishment to help with the repair of her bone
    tissue.

191.

192. It is said that 'milk is the perfect food'. This is because it contains all of the
essential food values except:
    A. Calcium
    B. Phosphorus
    C. Vitamin E
    D. Iron.

192.

193. If the correct answer to question 192 has been selected, which of the
following statements is true about this food factor.
    A. Babies are normally born with a sufficient reserve of this for the first two
    to three months of life
    B. It is not required by the body until the infant reaches six months of age
    C. It should be added to the baby's feeds once daily
    D. Babies do not require this particular food factor for the first three months
    of life as they have a natural immunity to infection.

193.

194. The normal fluid requirements for a baby of Tracey's birth weight are:
    A. 180 ml per kg body weight per 24 hours
    B. 150 ml per kg body weight per 24 hours
    C. 100 ml per kg body weight per 24 hours
    D. 50 ml per kg body weight per 24 hours.

194.

195. Tracey is now 4 weeks old and weighs 4 kg. Assuming that she has 5 feeds in 24 hours, her fluid requirement at each feed should be:
A. 180 ml
B. 150 ml
C. 120 ml
D. 100 ml

195.

One morning when Tracey was 4 weeks old, a health visitor called to see Mrs Lloyd and the baby. Mrs Lloyd welcomed the opportunity of being able to talk to her and ask advice on the care of Tracey.

---

196. The main aims of a health visitor's work are to:
A. Promote health and prevent disease
B. Provide information about social services and benefits which can be claimed
C. Provide nursing care for the very young and the elderly in their own homes
D. Prevent accidents by notifying the environmental health officer of any faulty heating, lighting or ventilation in the home.

196.

197. The health visitor's visit to Mrs Lloyd was to satisfy a legal requirement, because, in law a health visitor must visit:
A. Every household where there are children under the age of 5 years at least once a year
B. All babies during the first 6 weeks of life
C. Every woman during the first 8 weeks after a confinement
D. Every family which has a child with a congenital abnormality.

197.

198. The health visitor stressed to Mrs Lloyd the importance of keeping Tracey in the prone position when she was lying down. The term 'prone position' means lying:
A. Flat on the back
B. Flat on the front with the head turned to one side
C. In a crouched position with the hips and knees flexed
D. On the back with the hips flexed and abducted.

198.

199. Small babies must always be protected from the danger of an obstructed airway. All of the following points are important in the care of a baby, but which one must Tracey's mother be especially careful about when caring for her in the prone position?
   A. Breaking her wind after feeds
   B. Not placing a pillow under her head
   C. Ensuring that the bed clothes have been firmly tucked in at the sides
   D. Not placing the bed clothes any higher than shoulder level.

199.

200. In order to minimise the risk of suffocation which of the following items of clothing should never be worn by a small baby when left alone in the pram or cot?
   A. A nylon bib with plastic backing
   B. A woollen jacket with attached hood
   C. Plastic pants
   D. Mittens.

200.

Mrs Lloyd took the opportunity to ask the health visitor for advice about Tracey's vaccination programme. Both Mr and Mrs Lloyd had been feeling very concerned about this as they felt Tracey had enough problems with her hip condition, without having the extra discomfort of vaccinations.

201. Which of the following would be the most appropriate reply for the health visitor to make to Mrs Lloyd's enquiries?
   A. 'It would be better to wait until Tracey has her appointment at the hospital, and then you can ask the consultant about it'.
   B. 'Tracey really must have all her vaccinations as soon as possible, to help protect her from infection when she is admitted to hospital'.
   C. 'I think it would be wise to delay Tracey's vaccinations until after she has been into hospital, as she will have more resistance then'.
   D. 'It would be better for Tracey, if she followed the normal programme for vaccination as she needs all the help and protection we are able to give her'.

201.

202. When talking to the health visitor, Mrs Lloyd had expressed particular fears about the vaccination against whooping cough. She had heard that some babies suffered brain damage as a result of this injection.

   Whooping cough is caused by the:
   A. Coxsackie virus
   B. Haemolytic streptococcus
   C. Candida fungus
   D. Pertussis bacillus.

202.

203. In order to minimise the risk of brain damage, which of the following groups of children should never be given vaccination against whooping cough?

    Those who have a history of:
    A. Asthma
    B. Bronchitis
    C. Epilepsy
    D. Eczema.

203.

204. The purpose of vaccination is to provide a person with:
    A. Active artificially acquired immunity
    B. Passive artificially acquired immunity
    C. Active natural immunity
    D. Passive natural immunity.

204.

Tracey continued to progress well and when she was 4 months old her mother took her to the outpatient clinic for assessment of her hips. The orthopaedic surgeon was pleased with her progress and explained to Mrs Lloyd his plans for the management of Tracey over the next two years. The plan of management was to follow three stages:

1. Continue at home with double nappies and lying in the prone position until the age of 1 year, with regular hospital reviews.
2. At the age of 1 year admit to hospital for 3 weeks traction with increasing abduction followed by first stage surgery. Postoperative management would include 6 months splintage in abduction. Tracey would be at home for most of this time with regular hospital reviews.
3. At the age of 2 years, readmit to hospital for pelvic osteotomy. Postoperative management would include 6 weeks in a plaster hip spica, and again, Tracey would be nursed at home for most of this time.

205. Mrs Lloyd was pleased to know that Tracey would be able to spend much
     of her time at home, but expressed some fears about the hospital
     admissions. She could still remember her own lengthy treatment at the same
     hospital as Tracey was to be admitted to. Which of the following would
     provide the most reassurance to Mrs Lloyd?
     A. Tell her how much standards of care and treatment had improved in the
        past 20 years
     B. Give her a detailed explanation of how the various stages of treatment
        for Tracey differed from the treatment her mother had received
     C. Take her to the ward and let her meet the staff and see the cheerful
        ward environment
     D. Arrange for Tracey to be admitted to hospital for a few days 'trial period'
        so that she could get used to the nursing staff before being
        admitted for treatment.

                                                                           205.

206. When Tracey was a year old she was admitted to hospital for three weeks
     of gallows traction. (Ten days vertical followed by ten days increasing
     abduction.)
     With vertical gallows traction, counter traction is provided by:
     A. The weight of the child's body
     B. Elevating the foot of the bed
     C. Elevating the cross piece at the top of the frame
     D. The pressure of the bandages around the legs.

                                                                           206.

207. If gallows traction is to be effective, the baby must:
     A. not wear a napkin
     B. have bandages no higher than mid-thigh
     C. Have her buttocks raised above the level of the mattress
     D. Have her buttocks firmly resting on the mattress.

                                                                           207.

208. A baby nursed in a gallows abduction frame commonly has the head of the
     cot elevated. The purpose of this is to provide:
     A. Mental stimulus, by letting her have a better view of her surroundings
     B. Physical exercise, by letting her reach out for the traction cords
     C. An increased degree of traction
     D. An increased degree of counter traction

                                                                           208.

209. After 10 days of vertical traction, Tracey commenced increasing abduction
     of the hips for a further 10 days. At the final stage of reduction, the degree
     of abduction reached should be:
     A. 45°
     B. 90°
     C. 120°
     D. 180°.

                                                                           209.

Later that week Tracey was taken to the operating theatre for an examination under anaesthetic and arthrogram. The arthrogram showed that a limbus (fold of tissue) was preventing full reduction and it was necessary to operate to remove the limbus. Tracey then had a Lorenz (frog) plaster applied.

210. Tracey was normally a very active little girl. With reference to the activity of a child in a Lorenz plaster, which of the following statements is true?
   A. The child should be encouraged to be as active as her plaster permits
   B. The child should be allowed to move freely in her cot but should not be allowed to play on the floor
   C. Crawling is the only activity which should not be permitted
   D. The child should be given passive exercises of the shoulders, elbows and ankles every day.

210.

211. Four days later Mrs Lloyd was admitted to the mother and baby unit of the hospital to learn how to care for Tracey in her plaster before taking her home.

   With reference to the prognosis of a child with congenital dislocation of the hips, which of the following statements is true?
   A. The child is unlikely to ever attain a full range of movement of the hips without further dislocation taking place
   B. Children who are diagnosed in the first few weeks of life have a worse prognosis than those who are older before the first symptoms appear
   C. The older the child is when the diagnosis is made, the worse the prognosis
   D. The prognosis is good, only if the dislocation is so slight that it can be reduced by traction without open surgery.

211.

**Congenital dislocation of the hip answers and explanations
(Questions 180 to 211)**

True/false *(Page 21)*

180. **False**   Congenital dislocation of the hip is more common among girls than boys.

181. **False**   It is not uncommon for a woman who has had a congenital dislocation of the hip to have children with this disability.

182. **True**   There is often a history that the child was born in the breech position with the legs extended.

183. **False**   In this condition it is the acetabulum which is shallow, not the actual pelvis. If correctly treated, the hips should be stable by the time the individual reaches child bearing age.

184. **False**   The cause of congenital dislocation of the hip is unknown, although recent research indicates that there may be some link between this and an overproduction of female hormones. Note: Morbilli virus causes measles. German measles, which is known to damage the fetus is caused by the rubella virus.

185. **True**   Approximately two-thirds of all children with this disability have a unilateral dislocation.

186. **False**   The incidence of congenital dislocation of the hip is lower in the British Isles than in other parts of the world, notably northern Italy and Japan.

187. **False**   Every newborn baby is examined for the presence of congenital abnormalities, including dislocation of the hip.

Multiple choice *(Page 22)*

188. **A**   The baby's hips are gently manipulated in flexed abduction and may reveal a palpable 'click' as the head of the femur slips from the rim of the shallow acetabulum. This is known as a positive Ortolani sign. Trendelenburg sign (D) is also used in the diagnosis of congenital dislocation of the hip, but not for a baby of Tracey's age, as it involves standing on one leg!
Kernig's sign (B) is used in the detection of meningitis and Babinski's sign (C) indicates disease of the upper motor neurones. Note: dorsiflexion of the great toe (Babinski's sign) is normally exhibited by babies until they learn to walk.

189. **B** The purpose of treatment for congenital dislocation of the hips is to maintain the hips in abduction. In small babies this can be aided by the extra thickness provided by a double layer of napkins.

190. **D** Apart from her dislocated hips, Tracey is a normal healthy baby, and like all other babies she needs stimuli for healthy development, both mentally and physically. Mrs Lloyd should be encouraged to continue breast feeding Tracey as both mother and baby will benefit from the close contact. If Tracey is admitted to hospital while being breast fed (B) arrangements should be made for Mrs Lloyd to be admitted to the mother and baby unit, so that she can continue to feed Tracey.

191. **B** It is normal for babies to lose a little weight in the first few days of life and regain it by the time they are 10 days old. It has already been said that Tracey should develop normally and this includes her feeding regime, and weight gain (A, C and D).

192. **D** Milk is a good source of calcium, phosphorus and vitamin E; it does not contain iron.

193. **A** Babies are normally born with a sufficient reserve of iron for the first two to three months of life, and so do not need iron supplements in their diet. When mixed feeding is introduced (usually at about three months) foods containing iron are given.

194. **B** Babies of normal birth weight require a fluid intake of 150 ml per kg body weight per 24 hours. Premature babies require slightly more (180 ml per kg body weight per 24 hours).

195. **C** To calculate the fluid requirements for a baby's feed, multiply weight of baby by ml per kg per 24 hours and divide by number of feeds in 24 hours.

$$\frac{\text{Weight of Tracey (4 kg)} \times \text{ml per kg (150)}}{\text{Feeds in 24 hours (5)}} = x \text{ ml fluid}$$

$$\frac{4 \times \cancel{150}^{\,30}}{\cancel{5}_{\,1}} = 120 \text{ ml fluid}$$

196. **A** A health visitor may be called upon to provide information about social services (B), or to give advice on a wide range of subjects including safety in the home (D). By giving advice and information she fulfils the main aims of her rôle, which is to promote health and prevent disease. Although a health visitor is a registered nurse she does not normally provide nursing care (C) (although she may make arrangements for it's provision), unless she is employed in the dual rôle of health visitor and community sister.

197. **B** It is a legal requirement that every baby must be visited by a health visitor during the first six weeks of life (B). This gives her an opportunity to assess the baby's progress and also the progress of the mother.

198. **B** The prone position means lying flat on the front (B). Lying flat on the back (A) is the supine position. Babies normally adopt the crouched position (C) at about 6 months when preparing to crawl. Lying flat on the back with the hips flexed and abducted is the position in which the baby is examined for the presence of congenital dislocation of the hip (described in explanation to Question 188).

199. **B** A pillow should not be placed under the head of any small baby, but it is particularly important to avoid doing this if the baby is in the prone position, because of the risk of the baby's face being buried in the pillow, so causing suffocation.

200. **A** Plastic bibs of any type should not be worn by small babies because of the great risk that, while moving, the baby may place the plastic over the face and so suffocate. Plastic pants (C) will not be removed by a small baby, but caution is needed with older children. Woollen materials (B and D) are porous and so less dangerous than plastic.

201. **D** It has already been said that Tracey should be treated as a normal healthy baby as far as is practicable. She should follow the normal programme for vaccination, while care should be taken to plan her programme so that vaccinations do not coincide with proposed admissions to hospital. The success of 'community care' for any patient depends on team work, and the health visitor, family practitioner and consultant would all be involved in discussing and planning Tracey's care (A). It would cause Mrs Lloyd unnecessary worry to suggest that Tracey is going to be exposed to infection when she is admitted to hospital (B and C).

202. **D** Whooping cough is caused by the pertussis bacillus. The other options listed are each responsible for a wide variety of conditions including meningitis (A), sore throats (B) and thrush (C).

203. **C** Vaccination against whooping cough should not be given to a child who has a history of fits of any kind (C), because of the risk of increased brain damage. Children with eczema (D) should not be given vaccination against smallpox as it can produce a very serious generalised reaction known as vaccinia.

204. **A**   Immunity may be either: (1) natural, e.g. inborn, or (2) acquired, e.g. in later life.

Acquired immunity may be obtained either: (1) naturally, e.g. by exposure to the disease, or (2) artificially, e.g. by injection.

Artificially acquired immunity may be either: (1) active, e.g. by giving vaccine which causes the patient to produce his/her own antibodies, or (2) passive, e.g. by giving serum containing antibodies.

From this it can be seen that vaccination is a form of active artificially acquired immunity.

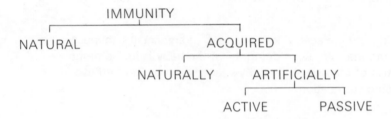

205. **C**   Mrs Lloyd's fears for Tracey are based on her own previous experiences. The best way of reassuring her is to let her see the ward and meet the staff. If she is able to see a bright cheerful ward, with children looking happy and well cared for, it will do more for her morale than simply to tell her about the changes that have taken place (A and B). A 'trial period' admission to hospital (D) is an unnecessary extravagance and may even do more harm than good.

206. **A**   With gallows traction, counter traction is provided by the weight of the
207. **C**   child's body (206A). This is why it is important for the buttocks to be
208. **A**   raised slightly above the surface of the mattress (207C). If the buttocks rest firmly on the mattress (207D) they take the weight of the body, so releasing counter traction and therefore making the traction ineffective. As far as the traction and counter traction are concerned it is not necessary to elevate either the head or the foot of the cot, but a baby lying flat on her back is unable to see around her. For this reason, the head of the cot is elevated, as it provides the baby with a better view of her surroundings (208A).

209. **D**   When reduction is complete the degree of abduction should be 180°

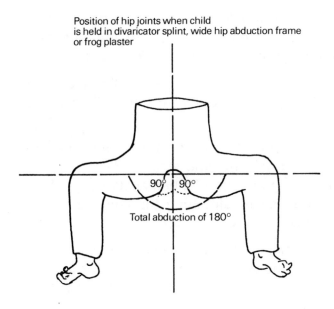

Position of hip joints when child
is held in divaricator splint, wide hip abduction frame
or frog plaster

90° | 90°

Total abduction of 180°

210. **A**   Children are very adaptable and quickly learn to become active despite
the confines of their plaster. This activity should be encouraged (A) and
special aids to mobility should be used when applicable (e.g. for the
older child, a low trolley on wheels, so that the child can propel herself
along the floor by using her arms and hands).

Note: because activity is encouraged, it is especially important for the
nurse to inspect the plaster regularly for signs of 'wear and tear' as a
weakened plaster will not be effective.

211. **C**   The earlier treatment is commenced, the greater the chance of success,
as normal growth and development is impeded until the femoral head is
reduced into the acetabulum. From this it can be seen that early
diagnosis is the key to success.

Fractured radius and ulna

The following questions (212–245) are based on, the case history given below:

It was a week before Christmas and Angela Roberts, aged 9 years, was very excited. Daddy had just come home with the Christmas tree and had said that Angela could help him to decorate it.

It was a big tree and Mr Roberts had to use a step ladder to arrange the lights on it. He then went out to the tool shed to put away the spare bulbs.

Angela's greatest wish was to put the fairy on top of the tree. Her father had told her she must not climb the step ladder but in her excitement she forgot his warning. She climbed to the top of the ladder, but still she could not reach. Clutching the fairy tightly she leant forward towards the tree...

Mrs Roberts was in the kitchen when she heard the crash. She rushed into the lounge and found Angela lying on the floor. Her left arm was twisted under her body, and the step ladder was lying across Angela's legs.

Matching item questions

The next 15 questions (212–226) are based on the cause, prevention and effects of accidents in varying situations, and are all of the matching item type. They consist of two lists. On the left is a list of lettered items (A, B, C etc.). On the right is a list of numbered items. Study the two lists and for each item in the numbered list select the appropriate item from the lettered list. You may indicate your answer by writing the appropriate letter in the right hand margin.

Note. There are more items in the lettered list than in the numbered lists and you will therefore not use all the items in the lettered list.

212–214. From the list on the left select the type of accident most likely to occur as a result of each situation on the right.

A. Burns	212. Children playing with empty bottles	212.
B. Scalds		
C. Poisoning	213. Babies playing with talcum powder container	213.
D. Cuts		
E. Choking.	214. Saucepan handles turned 'outwards' on the kitchen stove.	214.

215–217. From the list on the left select the situation most likely to cause each
incident on the right.

A. Loose slates on roof	215. Fire	215.
B. Electric flex tucked under carpet		
C. Thawing of frozen water pipes	216. Flood	216.
D. Worn tap washers		
E. Aerosol can on sunny window sill.	217. Explosion	217.

218–220. From the list on the left select the age group most commonly found to
sustain the injury on the right.

A. Small babies	218. Fractured shaft of femur	218.
B. Children		
C. Children and adults	219. Colles fracture	219.
D. Adults between 35–50 years		
E. Elderly people.	220. Supracondylar fracture of humerus.	220.

221–223. From the list on the left select the priority to match the list on the right,
when rendering first aid at the scene of an accident.

A. Arrest haemorrhage	221. 1st priority	221.
B. Observe for other injuries		
C. Maintain a clear airway	222. 2nd priority	222.
D. Prevent further accident		
E. Reassure the patient.	223. 3rd priority.	223.

224–226. From the list on the left select the first aid most applicable for the
injury on the right.

A. Immerse the injured part in cold water	224. Capillary haemorrhage	224.
B. Apply pressure directly over the injured part	225. Corrosive poisoning	225.
C. Apply hot compresses	226. Superficial burn.	226.
D. Give an emetic		
E. Give plenty of water orally		
F. Apply an alkali to the injured part.		

Fortunately Angela was fully conscious when her mother found her. Her left knee was very painful, she could not move it, but otherwise, apart from being very pale and frightened, she seemed unhurt. Mrs Roberts wrapped Angela in a blanket while her husband fetched the car. They then took Angela to the accident and emergency department of the local hospital. There it was found that she had sustained a greenstick fracture of the midshaft of the left radius and ulna.

Multiple choice questions
The following questions (227–245) are all of the multiple choice type. Questions 227–237 are based on various types of fracture, the others are based on this case history. Read the questions and from the possible answers select the ONE which you think is correct. You may indicate your answer by writing the appropriate number in the space provided or against the question number on your answer sheet.

227. A greenstick fracture is defined as one in which the: 227.
    A. Bone is bent, but there is no break in the continuity of the compact tissue or periosteum
    B. Bone is broken at one side and bent at the other
    C. Periosteum is completely severed, while the underlying compact tissue is unbroken.
    D. Periosteum and compact tissue are not broken but the underlying bone marrow is damaged.

228. Which of the following is associated with the greatest risk of damage to the brachial artery?   228.
    A. Dislocation of shoulder
    B. Dislocation of elbow
    C. Mid-shaft fracture of radius
    D. Supracondylar fracture of humerus.

229. A comminuted fracture is defined as one which always: 229.
    A. Communicates with an open wound
    B. Has the bone broken into more than two pieces
    C. Causes injury to the surrounding organs
    D. Has the fractured ends of the bone driven into each other.

230. A compression fracture would be most likely to occur in a: 230.
    A. Vertebra
    B. Scapula
    C. Patella
    D. Pelvis

231. Which of the following fractures is associated with the classic 'dinner fork' deformity?   231.
    A. Pott's
    B. Smith's
    C. Bennett's
    D. Colles.

232. Which of the following types of fracture is associated with the greatest risk of infection?
    A. Comminuted
    B. Compression
    C. Complicated
    D. Compound.

232.

233. Which of the following diseases is associated with the greatest risk of pathological fracture of the bone?
    A. Multiple sclerosis
    B. Rheumatoid arthritis
    C. Myasthenia gravis
    D. Paget's disease.

233.

234. A patient who sustains a fracture dislocation of the cervical spine will most probably experience:
    A. Hemiplegia
    B. Tetraplegia
    C. Monoplegia
    D. Paraplegia.

234.

235. Which of the following is most likely to be used for internal fixation of a fractured shaft of femur?
    A. Smith Peterson pin
    B. Kirschner wire
    C. Küntscher nail
    D. Steinmann pin.

235.

236. When nursing a child who has sustained a supracondylar fracture of humerus which of the following observations is it most important for the nurse to make regularly?
    A. Radial pulse on the injured arm
    B. Radial pulse on the unaffected arm
    C. Carotid pulse on the same side as the injury
    D. Any pulse which is easily accessible.

236.

237. If the correct answer to question 236 has been selected, the main reason why this observation is so important is because:
    A. An increase in pulse rate indicates that the brachial artery has been severed
    B. Absence of pulse indicates that the brachial artery has been trapped
    C. This type of fracture is associated with an especially high risk of pulmonary embolism
    D. A change in pulse rate and volume is usually the first indication of any change in the patient's general condition.

237.

After he had seen the X-rays, the casualty officer explained to Mr and Mrs Roberts that he would need their permission to set Angela's arm in a good position, and apply plaster of Paris. He also explained that in view of the fact that Angela had fallen from a height he would prefer to keep her in hospital overnight for observation, but providing there were no complications she could go home the following day.

238. Prior to having the plaster applied, Angela's arm was manipulated. In this situation, manipulation is a term which implies:
   A. An open surgical operation to ensure the bone fragments are in a good position and not trapping any nerves or blood vessels
   B. Movement of the fragments of the bone, at the fracture site, until they are in a good position for healing
   C. The insertion of 'guide wires' to ensure that the bone is in perfect alignment
   D. Violent, forceful movement of the injured arm to free the bone fragments from surrounding ligaments and so prevent adhesions.

238.

239. Bearing in mind what we know of Angela, which of the following observations would it be most important for the nurse to maintain accurately after Angela has been admitted to the children's ward?
   A. Temperature
   B. Blood pressure
   C. Power and movement of her lower limbs
   D. Size and reaction of her pupils.

239.

240. If the correct answer to question 239 has been selected, the reason why this observation is so important in Angela's case is because:
   A. Hypothermia is an early indication of cerebral anoxia
   B. Hypotension indicates an increase in the degree of shock
   C. Paralysis of the lower limbs may be the first indication of damage to the spinal cord
   D. Unequal pupils may indicate the presence of a cerebral haematoma.

240.

241. Which of the following is the most important feature in the drying of Angela's plaster cast?
   A. Avoid covering the plaster with plastic sheeting
   B. Apply plaster bending shears at the first sign of any swelling of the extremities
   C. When touching the plaster, use only the palms of the hands
   D. Avoid using any form of hot convection air currents.

241.

242. Applying direct radiant heat to a wet plaster must always be avoided. The main reason for this is because:
    A. A plaster that dries too quickly will not retain its shape
    B. The patient may be burnt through the plaster
    C. Heat may cause the plaster to shrink and become too tight
    D. Heat will cause the blood vessels to dilate and so increase the risk of oedema.

242.

243. If Angela complains of tingling and itching inside her plaster at a point level with the head of the ulna, which of the following explanations should the nurse suspect first?

    The symptoms are probably caused by:
    A. A perfectly natural return of sensation following the original injury
    B. The early stages of a pressure sore forming
    C. Damage to the peripheral sensory nerve supply
    D. The radial artery being trapped by the bone fragments.

243.

Happily Angela did not develop any complications during her night in hospital. The next day, Sister talked to Angela and her mother about the care of her plaster and gave Mrs Roberts a card with instructions written on it and an appointment for Angela to attend the fracture clinic.

Then Mrs Roberts took her daughter home, and to Angela's great delight her father had decorated the tree, and there at the very top was the fairy quite unharmed by the events of the previous day.

244. With reference to the healing of a fracture, which of the following statements is true?
    A. Callus formation is the first stage of repair
    B. The first stage of repair is haematoma formation, which is gradually replaced by granulation tissue
    C. A broken bone will eventually unite and and be restored to full function, but the torn periosteum will never repair
    D. Callus is not formed until after full ossification has taken place.

244.

245. With reference to the time taken for a fracture to heal, which of the following statements is most accurate?
    A. Impacted fractures unite more quickly than displaced fractures
    B. Spiral fractures take longer to unite than transverse fractures
    C. Fractures of the arm take longer to unite than similar type fractures of the leg
    D. Fractures which have not fully united after 4 months require a displacement osteotomy.

245.

Fractured radius and ulna answers and explanations
(Questions 212–245)

Matching item answers *(Page 34)*

212. **D**   Domestic accidents can happen very easily, especially when there are
213. **E**   young children or elderly people in the house. A child playing with an
214. **B**   empty bottle may fall causing the bottle to break. Serious injury may
result from this. Babies should never be allowed to play with talcum
powder containers, they tend to put all play things to the mouth and if
the lid should become loosened, inhalation of the powder would cause
the child to choke.

If saucepan handles are left turned 'outwards' on the stove a child may
pull at them and be scalded by the contents if the saucepan overturns.

215. **B**   If an electric flex is tucked under a carpet, it may become frayed by
216. **C**   friction and eventually cause a fire.
217. **E**   When water pipes are frozen they may crack as a result of expansion.
As the ice thaws water leaks through the cracks and causes flooding.

Aerosol cans carry a warning that they are pressurised and should not be
exposed to heat. For this reason they should not be left on a sunny
windowsill as glass reflects the sun and intensifies the heat.

218. **C**   Fractures of the shaft of femur are common in children and adults.
219. **E**   While Colles fracture is more common in elderly people, supracondylar
220. **B**   fracture of the humerus is more common in children.

221. **C**   When rendering first aid, the first priority is always to maintain a clear
222. **A**   airway. If this is not done, all other measures are pointless. Having
223. **D**   established that the airway is clear, the second priority is to arrest haemorrhage. It is also essential to prevent further accident, e.g. divert traffic.

224. **B**   Pressure applied directly over the injured part is usually effective in
arresting capillary haemorrhage (B).

225. **E**   When a corrosive poison has been taken plenty of water should be
given orally to dilute the poison (E). (Note: NEVER give an emetic, as
this will cause further damage to the alimentary canal as the corrosive
poison is vomited back and may also result in damage to the respiratory
tract due to inhalation of the vomit.) The patient should then be taken
to hospital as quickly as possible, where it may be considered necessary
to neutralise the poison. Acid poisons may be neutralised by giving an
alkali such as milk of magnesia. Alkali poisons may be neutralised by
giving an acid such as dilute vinegar. In either case a demulcent such
as white of egg may be given to soothe inflammation.

226. **A**   Superficial burns are best treated by immersing the part in cold water

Multiple choice answers *(Page 37)*

---

227. **B** The greenstick fracture, derives its name from the trees in spring when the sap is rising and the branches are supple. If you have ever tried to pick a spray of 'pussy willow' you may have found the twig snaps at the point of pressure, but remains securely hinged on one side. In the same way, children whose bones are young and pliant often sustain an incomplete, or 'greenstick' fracture.

228. **D** Supracondylar fracture of the humerus is an injury of the elbow. The great danger with this particular injury is that the brachial artery may become trapped (or subjected to friction) by displacement of the broken bone.

229. **B** A comminuted fracture is one in which the bone is broken into more than two pieces.

     A fracture which is associated with an open wound (A) is known as an 'open' or 'compound' fracture.

     A fracture which causes injury to surrounding organs (C) is known as a complicated fracture. When the fractured ends of a bone are driven into each other (D) it is known as an impacted fracture.

230. **A** Compression fractures most commonly occur in the vertebral column. As the name implies, the vertebrae are compressed or crushed together.

231. **D** The typical 'dinner fork' deformity is seen with Colles fracture (lower end of radius).

     Smith's fracture (B) also occurs at the lower end of the radius, but with displacement towards the palmar aspect, and is sometimes called reversed Colles fracture. Bennett's fracture (C) occurs at the thumb and Pott's fracture (A) occurs at the lower end of the fibula.

232. **D**   It has already been said that a compound fracture is one which is associated with an open wound. Our skin helps to protect us from harmful organisms, and whenever the skin surface is broken, there is a great risk of infection.

233. **D**   Paget's disease is a condition in which the bones are thin and brittle and therefore are particularly liable to fracture.
Multiple sclerosis and myasthenia gravis (A and C), are diseases affecting the nervous system. Rheumatoid arthritis (B) affects the joints.

234. **B**   When a patient sustains a fracture dislocation of the spine, any paralysis present will be below the point of injury. Therefore the higher the injury, the greater the area of paralysis. A patient with fracture of the cervical spine may be paralysed from the neck down and this is known as tetraplegia (or quadraplegia).

Hemiplegia (A) is paralysis of one side

Monoplegia (C) is paralysis of one limb.

Paraplegia (D) is paralysis of both lower limbs.

235. **C**   Internal fixation of a fractured shaft of femur may be achieved by use of an intramedullary nail (Küntscher nail). A Steinmann pin (D) and a Kirschner wire (B) may also be used for treatment of a fractured shaft of femur, but not for internal fixation. Their purpose would be to secure skeletal traction. A Smith Peterson pin (A) is used for a fractured neck of femur.

236. **A**   Supracondylar fracture of the humerus is an injury of the elbow, in
237. **B**   which there is a very great risk of the brachial artery becoming damaged by the displaced bone pieces. The brachial artery supplies the forearm and hand with oxygenated blood, and it is essential for this blood supply to be maintained. Therefore, it is vitally important that the nurse takes the radial pulse of the injured arm regularly, as a decrease in the volume will give an early indication of any damage to the brachial artery. She should also observe the circulatory return to the tips of the fingers after applying pressure.

238. **B**   A fracture may be reduced by open surgical operation (A) or by manipulation (closed reduction). This involves passive movement of the limb until the bone fragments at the fracture site are in a good position for healing (B). Violent forceful movement (D) should not be used because of the risk of damaging nerves and blood vessels. After manipulation an X-ray is taken to ensure that the bone is in a satisfactory position.

239. **D**   Angela fell from a ladder and although fully conscious it is possible that
240. **D**   she may have sustained a head injury. The purpose of her admission to
hospital would have been so that neurological observations could be
maintained regularly. These observations would include all the options
listed in question 239, but for Angela the most important observation
would be the size and reaction of her pupils, as unequal pupils may
indicate the presence of a cerebral haematoma. If this occurs, the
patient's condition will deteriorate as the haematoma causes pressure
on the brain. It is also important to observe her response to any
stimulus.

241. **A**   A plaster cast should be dried slowly by exposure to the air, and this
242. **B**   will take about 48 hours. During this time many points of nursing care
are important, but of the options listed, the most important is to avoid
covering the plaster with plastic sheeting, as this will retain the moisture
and increase heat. Never apply direct radiant heat to a wet plaster,
because apart from the risk of the plaster cracking there is a very great
danger of the patient being burnt through the plaster.

243. **B**   Nurses must always be alert for the possibility of a patient developing a
pressure sore inside a plaster cast. This risk is increased at any area
where there is a bone prominence. As with pressure sores in any other
area, a sensation of 'pins and needles' is often the first symptom.
Damage to the nerve supply (C) may be indicated by loss of sensation
in the fingers and damage of the blood supply (D) may be indicated by
the colour and temperature of the fingers.

244. **B**   When a bone breaks, it bleeds from the broken ends. This blood forms a
clot (haematoma) which holds the two broken ends together. Gradually
this is replaced by soft fibrous (granulation) tissue. The next stage of
repair is for the soft tissue to convert slowly to hard bone tissue
(callus).

245. **A**   Generally impacted fractures (bone ends driven into each other) unite
more quickly than displaced fractures. Spiral fractures unite more
quickly than transverse fractures (B), and fractures of the leg take
longer to unite than similar fractures of the arm (C). Many fractures will
take longer than four months to unite fully, without necessarily needing
further operative measures (D).

Meniscectomy

The following questions (246–266) are based on the case history given below:

Colin Reynolds, aged 19 years, was a student at university. He enjoyed most forms of sport, but his main interest was playing football. During the past year he had shown great talent for this sport and he was hoping eventually to become a professional player. Colin's greatest ambition was to play for England in a Cup Final.

Three months ago Colin received an injury to his left knee while playing in a charity match. The knee was very painful and swollen and the medical officer diagnosed a meniscus injury.

True/false questions

The following questions (246–266) consist of a number of statements, some of which are true and some of which are false. Consider each statement and decide whether you think it is true or false. You can indicate your answer by writing T for true or F for false in the right-hand margin beside each statement.

246. Cruciate ligament is another name for the meniscus.	246.
247. Men sustain a torn meniscus more frequently than women.	247.
248. Coal miners working in a squatting position are prone to injury to the meniscus.	248.
249. Tearing of the meniscus most commonly occurs when the knee is fully extended.	249.
250. A sudden twisting movement with the knee semi-flexed is a common cause of injury to the meniscus.	250.
251. Tears of the menisci commonly occur in footballers.	251.

Following the initial injury Colin had several episodes of severe pain in the knee associated with swelling. In view of this he was referred to the outpatient department of the local hospital for further investigations.

252. When a torn meniscus is suspected the immediate action for the first aider to take is to apply hot compresses to the injured knee.	252.

253. 'Locking' of the knee joint rarely accompanies tears of the meniscus.   253.

254. Following injury to the meniscus effusion of synovial fluid commonly   254.
     occurs, which prevents the patient from moving his knee.

255. An arthrotomy is a diagnostic procedure which involves injecting radio-   255.
     opaque dye into the knee joint.

256. Straight X-rays are normally adequate to demonstrate tears of the menisci.   256.

257. If locking of the knee joint occurs, emergency meniscectomy must be   257.
     performed within 24 hours.

Following investigation a diagnosis of torn left medial meniscus
was confirmed and arrangements were made for Colin's admission
to hospital for a meniscectomy.

258. When a meniscectomy is performed, both menisci are removed from the   258.
     affected leg, to give the joint greater stability.

259. Following a meniscectomy the patient is permanently unable to flex his   259.
     knee joint.

260. Postoperatively the knee is usually immobilised in a Thomas's splint, by   260.
     applying fixed skeletal traction.

261. Flexion of the knee must be prevented in the early postoperative period.   261.

262. In order to avoid making the patient too drowsy to co-operate with the   262.
     physiotherapist, postoperative analgesics should not be given for the first 24
     hours.

263. Active quadriceps exercises are an important feature in the postoperative   263.
     regime.

264. Straight-leg-raising with weights added to the foot is an effective way of   264.
     strengthening the quadriceps muscles.

265. Full flexion and extension of the knee joint is not possible after the   265.
     meniscus has been removed.

266. On discharge from hospital the patient should be told that he will be able to 266.
     play football again, when his leg has fully recovered.

Meniscectomy answers and explanations (questions 246–266)

---

246. **False** Another name for the meniscus is semilunar cartilage, because it is crescent-shaped. The cruciate ligaments are also in the knee joint, they connect the tibia to the femur.

247. **True** Injuries of the meniscus are far more common in men than in women, because of their occupations and sporting activities.

248. **True** Working in a crouched position with the knee flexed is a common cause of injury to the meniscus.

249. **False** Tearing of the meniscus occurs as a result of a sudden twisting
250. **True** movement with the knee flexed and the foot fixed to the ground.
251. **True** This action frequently takes place while playing football, which is why injury to the meniscus is so common among players.

252. **False** Heat would cause dilatation of the blood vessels, which would increase the degree of effusion. The correct procedure would be the application of a pressure bandage.

253. **False** 'Locking' of the knee joint frequently occurs when the meniscus is torn. The injury occurs when the knee is semi flexed, and the term 'locked knee' means that the patient is unable to extend his knee because the tear blocks free movement.

254. **True** Effusion (collection of synovial fluid) commonly occurs when the meniscus is torn. This causes the knee to become swollen and the patient is unable to move it.

255. **False** Arthrotomy means incision into a joint. The procedure described in this question is called an arthrography.

256. **False** Cartilage does not show up on straight X-rays.

257. **False** It is important for the effusion to subside before the patient has surgery. Next time you nurse a patient who has had a meniscectomy read his case notes. He will probably have been admitted from the waiting list with a history of injury some weeks before followed by a period of rest, with a pressure bandage applied to the knee.

258. **False** There is no point in removing a healthy meniscus from the knee.

259. **False** The purpose of performing a meniscectomy is to restore the knee joint to full function.

260. **False** The knee is usually immobilised in a plaster cylinder or pressure
261. **True** bandage in order to prevent flexion of the knee in the postoperative
period.

262. **False** While it is true that it is important for the patient to co-operate with
the physiotherapist, he will not be able to do so if he is in severe
pain.

263. **True** It is important for the patient to exercise his thigh muscles
(quadriceps) regularly. This must be done for five minutes once
every hour, the nurse encouraging the patient in the absence of the
physiotherapist.

264. **True** The weights increase the effort needed to extend the knee.

265. **False** In time the knee should be capable of a full range of movement. The
266. **True** patient will find it reassuring to know this when he leaves hospital,
but it should be stressed that he should not engage in active sport
immediately and his progress will be assessed at the outpatient
clinic. Many professional footballers have had one or more cartilages
removed from their knees.

Mid-shaft fracture of the femur

The following questions (267–280) are based on the case history given below:

Janice Jones is a 19-year-old student nurse in her second year of training. While visiting her parents for her off duty, Janice was involved in a motor cycle accident and sustained a mid-shaft fracture of her right femur. Subsequently, Janice was admitted via the accident and emergency department to a local hospital, where fixed skeletal traction was applied, and her injured leg was placed in a Thomas's splint.

Multiple choice questions

The following questions (267–280) are all of the multiple choice type. Read the questions and from the possible answers select the ONE which you think is correct. You may indicate your answer by writing the appropriate number in the space provided or against the question number on your answer sheet.

267. Which of the following would be suitable to use for applying traction to Janice's leg?
   A. Küntscher nail
   B. Steinmann pin
   C. Rush nail
   D. McLoughlin nail-plate.

| 267. |

268. Skeletal traction is best defined as:
   A. Any form of traction other than that applied directly to the skin
   B. Any form of traction which does not involve the use of weights and pulleys
   C. A form of traction which is always used in conjunction with an intramedullary nail
   D. Traction which is always applied directly to the bone.

| 268. |

269. With reference to skeletal traction which of the following statements is true?
   A. This traction is only effective when used in conjunction with a Thomas' splint
   B. Greater traction can be applied by using this method then by using skin traction
   C. In order that this traction may be effective the patient must remain in the recumbent position
   D. With this method of traction there is less risk of complications occurring than with other types.

| 269. |

270. With reference to fixed traction which of the following statements is true?
   A. No weights or pulleys are used for this form of traction
   B. An abduction frame must always be used in conjunction with this form of traction
   C. Injuries of the femur are the only conditions which can be effectively treated by this form of traction
   D. Fractures treated by this method heal more quickly than those treated with sliding or balanced traction.

   270.

271. When fixed traction is applied, countertraction is supplied by:
   A. The weight of the patient's body
   B. Tying the cords from the U-loop or stirrup to the end of the splint
   C. Elevating the foot of the bed
   D. Suspending the Thomas' splint from the Balkan beam.

   271.

272. When fixed traction is applied the degree of traction is increased by:
   A. Attaching a weight to the bottom of the splint
   B. Attaching a weight to the top of the splint
   C. Tightening the traction cords
   D. Loosening the traction cords.

   272.

Apart from the routine general nursing care of Janice, it was important for the nursing staff to pay special attention to observing the state of her traction each day. Her leg and splint were checked daily, and any necessary adjustments made.

273. Which of the following did the nursing staff need to be particularly careful about when caring for Janice?
   A. 'Boosting' her general morale
   B. Keeping the ring of the splint well padded
   C. Keeping her toenails short
   D. Cleanliness around the pin track.

   273.

274. When caring for Janice which of the following tasks must the nursing staff never perform without the permission of the doctor?
   A. Tightening the slings of the splint
   B. Abducting the limb
   C. Medially rotating the limb
   D. Retying the knots of the traction cord.

   274.

275. The slings of a Thomas' splint are secured by means of kilt pins, or some similar device. These are always secured on the lateral aspect of the splint. The main reason for this position is to:
A. Prevent friction against the other leg
B. Increase the degree of medial rotation
C. Provide more support for the leg
D. Provide easy access for the nursing staff.

275.

276. All of the following are important pressure points. Which should the nursing staff be especially careful to observe for signs of soreness when caring for Janice?
A. Malleoli
B. Groin
C. Sacrum
D. Shoulders.

276.

277. Sometimes patients with fixed traction have the end of the splint secured to the bed end, and the foot of the bed elevated. The purpose of this is to:
A. Relieve pressure around the ring of the splint
B. Provide a greater degree of countertraction
C. Ensure abduction is maintained
D. Allow greater flexion of the knee.

277.

278. When fixed traction is in use, which of the following is likely to be the first indication that too great a force is being exerted?
A. The patient complains of pain in the calf
B. The traction cord starts to fray
C. The pin starts to bend
D. The patient slips down the bed.

278.

279. The greatest danger to the patient as a result of having skeletal traction is:
A. Infection of the pin track
B. A residual sinus left by the pin track
C. Depression of the bone marrow
D. Damage to the periosteum.

279.

280 The main difference between fixed and sliding (or balanced) traction is that with fixed traction:
A. It is not possible to use elastoplast or ventfoam extensions
B. The nurse must be especially careful not to interrupt the degree of traction when lifting the patient
C. The patient may be safely transported from her bed to a chair or trolley without any interference to the degree of traction
D. It is necessary to maintain the traction for a longer period of time.

280.

Janice made a good recovery and was discharged from hospital 14 weeks later.

Mid-shaft fracture of the femur answers and explanations
(Questions 267–280)

267. **B**   A Steinmann pin is used for applying skeletal traction. It is driven through the upper end of the tibia, and a stirrup or U-loop is attached. Küntscher nails (A) and Rush nails (C) are both used in the treatment of fractured shaft of femur, but they are intramedullary nails used for internal fixation of the fracture. A McLoughlin nailplate is used for internal fixation of a fractured neck of femur.

268. **D**   Skeletal traction is always applied directly to the bone. This may be to the tibia, as in Janice's case, or to the skull for treatment of an injury to the cervical spine. Skeletal traction may be either 'fixed' or 'sliding' (balanced). If you answered (A) to this question, remember that apart from skin traction and skeletal traction, there is also a third type known as pulp traction.

269. **B**   Greater traction can be applied by this method because it is applied directly to the bone. Skeletal traction need not be used in conjunction with a Thomas' splint unless the traction is to be of the 'fixed' type (A). The position of the patient will vary according to the reason for the traction being applied (C), e.g. supine for skull traction. All patients confined to bed for any length of time are liable to develop complications of bed rest (e.g. pressure sores).

270. **A** The term 'fixed traction' means that traction is applied between two
271. **B** fixed points, no weights and pulleys are required. In this instance, the
272. **C** fixed points are:

1. The ring of the Thomas' splint against the ischial tuberosity in the groin.
2. The cord which attaches the U-loop to the end of the splint.

As the traction cord is tightened the amount of pull is increased, and at the same time the ring of the splint moves further up into the groin, and presses on the ischial tuberosity, so increasing the degree of counter traction. A 'T' piece or spigot may be used to maintain the tension of the traction cords if permitted.

FIXED TRACTION
Traction on that part of the limb between two fixed points

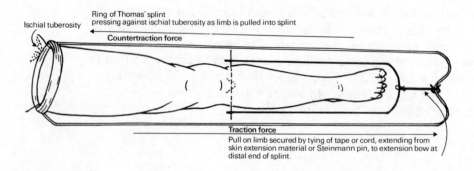

273. **D** Of the options listed A and C are important in the care of a patient, but because Janice has skeletal traction it is essential that the skin around the pin track is kept clean (D). (Remember that the pin passes through the bone and could be a source of infection if not kept clean). The ring of the Thomas' splint (B) is already padded and should fit accurately. Further padding will only cause pressure.

274. **D** When caring for Janice, it should be part of the daily routine to check the slings of the splint and adjust them if necessary (A). It may be necessary to abduct the limb slightly (B) to ease pressure around the ring of the splint. If the limb is laterally rotated, this should also be adjusted (C). However a nurse should not retie the knots of the traction cords if fixed traction is in use, unless permission is given, as the tightness of the tying affects the degree of traction.

275. **D**   Because the slings need to be adjusted daily, it is necessary for the nursing staff to have easy access to the kilt pins. If the kilt pins were applied medially, the nurse would have to lean across the patient's other leg. This would not only be uncomfortable for both the patient and the nurse, but would also make it difficult for the nurse to achieve the correct degree of tension on the slings.

276. **B**   It has already been said that as fixed traction is applied, counter traction is supplied by the splint moving further up the leg. As the degree of traction is increased the ring of the Thomas' splint often causes friction and pressure in the groin, and this area becomes likely to develop sores.

277. **A**   If a weight is tied to the foot of the splint and the foot of the bed is elevated, the splint will ease away from the groin slightly and so relieve the pressure. The greater the amount of traction applied, the greater is the risk of the groin becoming sore.

278. **C**   If the Steinmann pin should start to bend, it is a sign that too much traction is being applied.

279. **A**   If the surrounding skin is not kept clean, there is great danger of the pin track becoming infected (A). Provided the area is kept free of infection, the track normally heals quite quickly after the pin has been removed, without causing any residual damage to the bone structure (B, C and D).

280. **C**   Fixed traction has the disadvantage of increased pressure in the groin, but the great advantage to this form of traction is that, because it is between two fixed points, the patient may be safely moved without any interference to the degree of traction. Naturally, the nurse must be careful and ensure that the limb is always well supported. When sliding or balanced traction is in use, there is a greater risk that the degree of traction may be interrupted during routine nursing procedures, because it is dependent on the pull of the weights and these may easily become 'caught' on the bed rail, or lodged on the floor.

BALANCED OR SLIDING TRACTION
Traction on that part of the limb between two mobile points

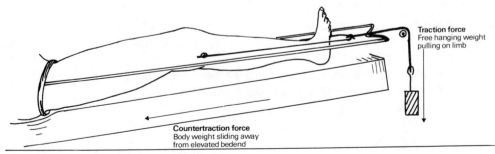

Traction force
Free hanging weight
pulling on limb

Countertraction force
Body weight sliding away
from elevated bedend

Fractured femur

The following questions (281–340) are based on the case history given below:

Miss Maggs, a spinster aged 70 years, lived alone in a small cottage which she had inherited from her mother 10 years ago. The cottage was old, rather isolated and situated 5 miles from the town. She was a keen gardener and spent much of her time out of doors or working in her greenhouse. Having lived there all her life she was not keen to move to a less isolated house.

Her sole companion was Minnie, a much loved and very pampered Persian cat. Minnie always had the cream of the milk for breakfast. She was large and had a beautiful glossy coat, while her mistress was small and thin! Miss Maggs always attributed her slight build to living an active life.

Miss Maggs had only one relative, a niece named Alice, who lived 200 miles away and who seldom saw her aunt.

One Friday morning, as was her usual custom, Miss Maggs went to town for her pension. She had never enjoyed crowded places and decided to walk in the park until it was time to return home. She was admiring the autumn colours when a passing cyclist swerved in front of her. While attempting to avoid the bicycle, Miss Maggs slipped on the fallen leaves and fell, landing heavily on her left side. It all happened so suddenly that she could not think what she was doing lying there on the ground. She was aware of terrible pain in her left leg and was unable to move it.

Multiple choice questions
The following questions (281–340) are all of the multiple choice type. Read the questions and from the possible answers select the ONE which you think is correct. You may indicate your answer by writing the appropriate number in the space provided or against the question number on your answer sheet.

281. Having sent someone to telephone for an ambulance, which of the following should be the first action of the person finding Miss Maggs?
    A. Cover her with his coat or jacket
    B. Ensure that too many people do not crowd around her
    C. Take the name and address of any witness to the accident
    D. Ascertain her identity.

281.

282. Having dealt with the four points listed in question 281 in their order of priority, the next important action to take would be to:
    A. Give her a warm sweet drink
    B. Carry her to the nearby sports pavilion
    C. Apply a temporary splint to the leg
    D. Look for other injuries.

282.

283. Miss Maggs was in a state of shock. This would be evident by:
    A. Rapid pulse and hot flushed face
    B. Rapid pulse and cold clammy skin
    C. Slow pulse and cold clammy skin
    D. Slow pulse and hot flushed face.

283.

284. In the case of Miss Maggs the shock would be classified as:
    A. Haemorrhagic and emotional
    B. Emotional and surgical
    C. Surgical and haemorrhagic
    D. Traumatic and emotional.

284.

In due course an ambulance arrived and Miss Maggs was taken to the accident and emergency department of the local hospital.

285. When Miss Maggs arrived at the accident and emergency department, the immediate priority of the nursing staff would be to provide reassurance and:
    A. Remove her splint in preparation for an X-ray to be taken
    B. Administer an analgesic
    C. Remove her clothes and observe for any external wounds
    D. Take and record her blood pressure.

285.

286. Which of the following actions of the nurse is likely to be most reassuring to Miss Maggs?
    A. Holding her hand and looking at her when speaking to her
    B. Asking the police to take a message to her next of kin
    C. Taking safe custory of her pension money and providing a receipt for it
    D. Folding her clothes carefully before putting them away.

286.

287. Which of the following is likely to cause greatest worry to Miss Maggs as a result of her accident?
    A. Being among strange people
    B. Being confined to bed
    C. The care of her garden
    D. The care of Minnie, her cat.

287.

In accordance with the Road Traffic Act 1972 the law provides for certain people attending an accident and emergency department to be charged a small fee.

288. With reference to this Act, which of the following statements is completely accurate?
    A. Every person requiring an ambulance as a result of an accident on the highway or in public grounds will be charged this fee
    B. The fee is only charged to people involved in an accident as a result of careless driving or where the alcohol level of the blood is above a certain limit
    C. The fee is charged to every person involved in an accident with a moving vehicle, either on the highway or in private grounds
    D. Every person involved in an accident with an insurable vehicle on the highway is liable to be charged the fee.

288.

289. This fee is charged to provide payment for the:
    A. Upkeep and maintenance of roads
    B. Upkeep and maintenance of ambulances
    C. Services of the first doctor attending the patient
    D. Services of the first police officer attending the scene of the accident.

289.

290. Although the law provides for certain people to be charged this fee, Miss Maggs would not have received a bill for her attendance at the department. This was because:
    A. People of retirement age are always exempt from payment
    B. Her accident did not involve a motor vehicle
    C. The cyclist causing the accident would have been responsible for payment
    D. There were no independent witnesses to the accident.

290.

After Miss Maggs had been examined by the doctor she was taken to the X-ray department where it was confirmed that she had sustained a fracture of her left femur.

291. Many different terms are used when describing fractures. With reference to this, which of the following statements is true?
   A. A fracture of the bone is always more serious than a broken bone
   B. A fracture of the bone always indicates involvement of surrounding structures, while the term broken bone indicates that there has been no involvement of nerves and blood vessels
   C. The terms 'fracture' and 'broken' both mean exactly the same
   D. The term broken bone always means a clean break into two or more pieces, while a fracture is a term used to indicate an incomplete break.

291.

Femur showing fracture site

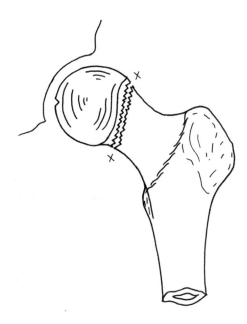

The next five questions relate to the diagram above.

292. On the diagram X marks the line of Miss Maggs's fracture. Fractures in this area of the femur are said to be:
   A. Intertrochanteric
   B. Subtrochanteric
   C. Intracapsular
   D. Extracapsular.

292.

293 Another way of describing this injury is to say that it is a fracture of the | 293.
femoral:
A. Head
B. Neck
C. Shaft
D. Tuberosity.

294. Elderly ladies commonly fracture the femur at this site after comparatively | 294.
minor injury. The most common contributory cause is:
A. Osteomyelitis
B. Osteoporosis
C. Paget's disease
D. Parkinson's disease.

295. Fractures at this site frequently result in a reduction of the blood supply to | 295.
which one of the following parts of the femur?
A. Shaft
B. Greater trochanter
C. Lesser trochanter
D. Head.

296. Which of the following treatments would Miss Maggs be most likely to | 296.
receive during her first 10 days in hospital?
A. Skin traction, internal fixation and plaster of Paris
B. Skin traction, internal fixation and physiotherapy
C. Skeletal traction, plaster of Paris and occupational therapy
D. Skeletal traction, physiotherapy and occupational therapy.

Once a clear diagnosis had been made Miss Maggs was admitted
to the female orthopaedic ward.

297. When preparing the bed for Miss Maggs's admission, which of the | 297.
following accessories would it be most important to have in position?
A. Bed cradle
B. Bed blocks
C. Overhead beam support (Balkan beam)
D. Rigid mattress support.

298. On admission to the ward Miss Maggs would most probably be nursed in | 298.
which of the following positions?
A. Upright
B. Prone
C. Semirecumbent
D. Left lateral.

299. If the correct answer has been selected in question 298, the reason for this | 299.
position would be to:
A. Prevent hypostatic pneumonia
B. Assist in preventing pressure sores due to friction
C. Prevent pain
D. Provide maximum support for the injured limb.

When Miss Maggs was settled into the ward, the doctor visited her and explained that she would need an operation to 'mend' her broken hip. The operation would take place the next day, but in the meantime the nurses were going to make her leg more comfortable.

The doctor then asked the ward sister to arrange for Miss Maggs to have traction applied to her injured limb with 2.5 kg weight.

300. Miss Maggs was to have her operation on the day after admission to | 300.
hospital. The most probable reason for this delay was to allow:
A. Callus formation to take place
B. The torn periosteum to repair
C. Her general condition to improve
D. Time to locate her next of kin.

301. Which of the following statements most aptly describes Pugh traction? It is: | 301.
A. A simple form of balanced skin traction
B. A special type of fixed traction
C. Only effective when used in conjunction with a Thomas' splint
D. Another name for Hamilton Russell traction.

302 Bearing in mind what we know of Miss Maggs, the most suitable way of | 302.
applying her traction would be by using:
A. A Steinmann pin
B. A Denham pin
C. Elastoplast extensions
D. Ventfoam extensions.

303. Which of the following would be the most likely position for Miss Maggs's | 303.
leg to be prior to having the traction applied?
A. Internally rotated and adducted
B. Internally rotated and abducted
C. Laterally (externally) rotated and adducted
D. Laterally rotated and abducted.

304. When applying a bandage over ventfoam traction, the most important rule for the nurse to remember is that the: | 304.
    A. 'Figure of eight' method is used
    B. Bandage is applied from ankle to groin
    C. Bandage is applied with even pressure
    D. Malleoli are protected from pressure.

305. When her traction had been secured, the foot of Miss Maggs's bed was elevated. The reason for this was to: | 305.
    A. Reduce the effects of shock
    B. Provide countertraction
    C. Prevent the weight touching the floor when the traction cord stretched
    D. Reduce oedema.

Despite the fact that her leg was now feeling more comfortable, Miss Maggs was very distressed and kept asking to go home. In due course the medical social worker came to see her.

306. The main purpose of the medical social worker's visit was most probably to: | 306.
    A. Complete the necessary forms for Miss Maggs's cottage to be adapted in preparation for her return home ·
    B. Obtain the key of the cottage in order to feed Minnie
    C. Obtain details of Miss Maggs's pension number in order to notify the Department of Health and Social Security of her admission
    D. Assess the general situation and decide what immediate help was needed.

307. Rehabilitation of Miss Maggs should commence: | 307.
    A. As soon as she is admitted to hospital
    B. Immediately she is allowed out of bed
    C. When she is allowed to weight-bear on her injured leg
    D. As soon as she can walk without aid.

308. With regard to the care of Minnie (the cat), which of the following would be the most appropriate action for the medical social worker to advise? | 308.
    A. Place Minnie in the care of a Private Cat's Home where she would have every care and attention
    B. Ask the local veterinary surgeon if Minnie could be resident at his surgery until her mistress returns home
    C. Ask the RSPCA if they would give her a temporary lodging home.
    D. Arrange to have her 'put to sleep' rather than let her pine for her mistress.

309. With regard to Miss Maggs's Department of Health and Social Security pension, which of the following statements is true?
    A. Admission to hospital never affects an entitlement to this pension
    B. Only patients admitted for long-term treatment in a psychiatric hospital are liable to have their pension reduced
    C. The pension is normally reduced by 25 per cent when a patient is admitted to hospital
    D. The pension is likely to be reduced when a patient stays in hospital longer than eight weeks.

309.

While the medical social worker was with Miss Maggs, the ward sister received a telephone call from a local press reporter. He was writing an account of the accident and wished to know how Miss Maggs was progressing.

---

310. Which of the following would be the most appropriate reply for the ward sister to give?
    A. 'She is as comfortable as can be expected'
    B. 'Hold the line please, while I ask if she minds letting me give you this information'
    C. 'I am sorry but I cannot give you that information. If you would like to hold the line I will transfer your call to the hospital administrator'
    D. 'I am sorry, but the medical social worker is with her at present. Would you phone back later when I have had an opportunity to speak to Miss Maggs?'

310.

311. Later that evening a junior nurse was serving hot drinks when Miss Maggs asked her to witness a Will she had made. In law a Will is only valid if it has been witnessed by:
    A. A solicitor and one other person
    B. A solicitor, or bank manager, or priest and one other person
    C. The chief beneficiary and one other person
    D. Any two independent people who are not beneficiaries.

311.

312. The law does not prevent nursing staff witnessing a patient's Will, but hospital authorities do not usually encourage the practice. The main reason for this is:
    A. The nurse may not be aware of circumstances in the family background of the patient which could lead to the Will being contested in Court
    B. As a safeguard against it being contested a Will must always be written in strictly legal terms which the nurse may not understand
    C. If the Will is contested, the nurse may be asked to testify in Court
    D. If the hospital or any of its staff were named as beneficiaries the Will would automatically become invalid on the grounds of coercion.

312.

313. Miss Maggs was particularly liable to develop pressure sores. The main   313.
     contributory factor to this was her:
     A. Slight build
     B. Lack of adequate diet
     C. State of shock
     D. Immobility.

314. Which of the following would be the best form of movement to prevent   314.
     Miss Maggs developing pressure sores?
     A. Give her passive limb movements for five minutes of each hour
     B. Alternate her position between supine and prone at two-hourly intervals
     C. Nurse her in the lateral position, alternating sides at two-hourly intervals
     D. Encourage and assist her to raise her buttocks frequently from the bed
        with the help of her trapeze ('monkey pole').

315. Which one of the following 'anti-pressure' devices would be most suitable   315.
     to use for Miss Maggs?
     A. A water bed
     B. A Stryker frame
     C. A full-length sheepskin
     D. An air ring.

316. Apart from movement and the use of anti-pressure devices, the most   316.
     important duty of the nurse in preventing Miss Maggs from developing
     pressure sores is to:
     A. Keep the skin clean and dry
     B. Massage the pressure area with spirit and talcum powder
     C. Ensure that she receives a good fluid intake
     D. Ensure that she is kept free of pain.

This was the first time Miss Maggs had experienced being a patient in hospital. When the bedpan was brought Miss Maggs was very apprehensive and although she needed to pass urine she told the nurse to take it away. Later she asked if she could get out of bed and go to the toilet.

317. When reassuring Miss Maggs which of the following would be the most appropriate answer for the nurse to give?
    A. 'I'm sorry Miss Maggs, but you may not get up because your leg is tied to the bed, I will bring you a bed pan'
    B. 'I'm sorry Miss Maggs, but you cannot walk on your leg because it is broken. Nurse and I will be very gentle when we lift you onto the bed pan'
    C. 'The doctor would like a sample of your water Miss Maggs, so it is best to use the bed pan just for this time'
    D. 'Just try to use the bedpan Miss Maggs and don't worry about the mess because we are used to it.'

318. With reference to placing Miss Maggs on a bed pan, which of the following statements is true?
    A. It is not necessary to warm the bed pan as Miss Maggs will be protected from direct contact with it by the bandages securing her traction
    B. When a patient has a fractured neck of femur, it is best to lift her no higher than five centimetres above the mattress and then gently push the bed pan into position
    C. Despite the fact that Miss Maggs will find it painful to be moved it is essential to reassure her and gain her co-operation
    D. Ideally, blankets should always be removed from the bed before lifting the patient, to prevent them resting on the traction cords.

319. With reference to the possible effects of placing Miss Maggs on a bed pan which of the following statements is true?
    A. Contaminated bed pans are the most common cause of urinary tract infection
    B. Releasing the pull of traction prior to lifting Miss Maggs will reduce the risk of dislocating her hip joint
    C. Improper positioning of a bed pan is a common contributory factor to pressure sores
    D. Movement of the injured leg increases the risk of deep vein thrombosis.

317.

318.

319.

320. Miss Maggs had a bowel action while on the bed pan. The junior nurses attending her were uncertain of the best way to clean her. With reference to this problem, which of the following statements is true?
    A. Under no circumstances must Miss Maggs be turned onto either side, as this could cause the bone fragments to dislocate
    B. Miss Maggs may be turned onto the unaffected side but not onto the injured side as this could cause a nerve to be trapped by the bone fragments
    C. Miss Maggs may be rolled onto the injured side but not onto the unaffected side as this would increase the degree of abduction
    D. With care the nurses may roll Miss Maggs onto either side without causing further injury.

320.

321. If Miss Maggs were to become restless during the night, which of the following would be the best way of ensuring her safety?
    A. Place cot sides in position to prevent her falling out of bed
    B. Lower the foot of her bed
    C. Ensure that she is given her prescribed sedation
    D. Ascertain the cause and act accordingly.

321.

At 10 p.m. the night staff received a telephone message from Miss Maggs's niece (Alice). Alice said she would arrive the next day to collect Minnie from her temporary lodging and take her back to the cottage. Alice would then stay on at the cottage until her Aunt was fit to return home.

Miss Maggs was very cheered by this news and had a fairly restful night.

Next morning the medical staff were pleased with her general condition and agreed to continue with surgery as planned, for reduction and internal fixation of the fracture.

322. Which of the following is most likely to be used for internal fixation of Miss Maggs's fracture?
    A. A nailplate
    B. Femoral head prosthesis
    C. Intramedullary nail
    D. Steinmann pin.

322.

323. When preparing Miss Maggs for theatre which of the following should the nurse do first?
   A. Check that her identiband is in position
   B. Give the prescribed premedication
   C. Ensure that she empties her bladder
   D. Remove the traction.

   323.

324. It is important for Miss Maggs to empty her bladder before having her operation because:
   A. This will prevent post-operative retention
   B. The bladder sphincter will relax during the anaesthetic
   C. Her full bladder may obstruct the surgeon's view of the fracture site
   D. Her full bladder would make her restless during the anaesthetic.

   324.

325. Another important aspect of preoperative care is to ensure that the patient does not have food or drink for a certain period before surgery. In Miss Maggs's case the minimum time for withholding oral fluids would be:
   A. 4 hours
   B. 6 hours
   C. 8 hours
   D. 12 hours.

   325.

326. By withholding food from Miss Maggs prior to surgery it is ensured that there is no food residue in the:
   A. Stomach only
   B. Stomach and duodenum only
   C. Stomach and small intestine only
   D. Whole of the gastrointestinal tract.

   326.

327. During this preparation period Miss Maggs became very thirsty and kept asking for a drink. Which of the following would be the most suitable answer for the nurse to give?
   A. 'I'm sorry Miss Maggs, but the doctors do not want you to have a drink and if I go against their wishes I shall get into trouble.'
   B. 'Just relax Miss Maggs and try to go to sleep, then you won't notice the thirst.'
   C. 'I'm sorry Miss Maggs, but I can't give you a drink because you are going to have an anaesthetic.'
   D. 'Not just now, dear, but as soon as you wake up from your operation you can have one.'

   327.

328. If, while sister is at lunch, the student nurse who is temporarily in charge of the ward finds another patient has given a drink to Miss Maggs, the first action of the nurse should be to:
   A. Notify the anaesthetist
   B. Telephone sister and tell her what has happened
   C. Pass a nasogastric tube and aspirate
   D. Stay with Miss Maggs and reassure her until sister returns.

   328.

Miss Maggs was given her prescribed premedication of pethidine 50 mg with atropine sulphate 0.6 mg at 1 p.m., and at 2 p.m. the porter came to take her to theatre.

329. How many microgrammes are equal to 0.6 milligrammes?
   A. 6
   B. 60
   C. 600
   D. 6000.

329.

330. The main purpose of giving atropine as a premedication is to:
   A. Hasten the action of the pethidine
   B. Minimise the side-effects of the pethidine
   C. Reduce bronchial secretions
   D. Stimulate the respiratory centre.

330.

331. In order to protect herself from possible effects of the drug which of the following must the nurse be especially careful to do when preparing an injection of atropine?
   A. Wear a mask
   B. Wear rubber gloves
   C. Cover the tip of the needle while expelling air from the syringe
   D. Use a wide-bore needle to draw up the solution.

331.

332. Having given the premedication to Miss Maggs the nurse must:
   A. Draw the curtains round the bed and leave the patient to sleep
   B. Keep her under close observation
   C. Check her identiband
   D. Put on her operation gown.

332.

In due course the theatre staff telephoned to say that Miss Maggs was ready to return to the ward. Staff nurse went to the theatre to collect Miss Maggs and took with her a junior nurse in order to teach her the procedure for escorting a patient from theatre. In this particular hospital, the procedure was for ward staff to report to the theatre staff stating the ward and name of the patient before going through to the recovery room to take custody of the patient.

333. Before taking custody of Miss Maggs the ward nurse must ensure that:
    A. She knows what operation has been performed
    B. A postoperative drug has been written on the treatment sheet
    C. She knows if the patient has any wound drainage
    D. She collects the X-rays.

333.

334. Before leaving theatre, staff nurse must attend to all the following duties, but which must be her final action before actually wheeling Miss Maggs out of the recovery room?
    A. Ensure the patient is adequately covered with blankets
    B. Satisfy herself that there is sufficient fluid in the intravenous bag to last until they arrive at the ward.
    C. Satisfy herself that the patient is in a fit condition for the journey
    D. Check the position of the patient's limbs, to ensure that the circulation is not impaired by pressure.

334.

335. Sometimes it is necessary to take patients to the ward while they are still unconscious. With reference to this which of the following statements is true?
    A. Danger of the patient's airway becoming blocked is eliminated if an artificial pharyngeal airway is used.
    B. If the patient's airway is completely blocked the nurse must administer oxygen immediately
    C. The patient's jaw should be held well forward to prevent the tongue slipping back
    D. A cuffed endotracheal tube must always be in position before the patient is moved.

335.

Miss Maggs arrived at the ward safely and was put into bed. She had had an internal fixation of her fracture by means of a pin and plate, consequently she did not need to have traction after surgery. The surgeon had prescribed a post operative drug of 'Pethidine 50 mg 4-hrly.'

336. Which of the following statements is true regarding the safe-keeping of pethidine in hospital?
    A. It must be stored in a specially coloured container
    B. It must be stored in the 'Poisons' cupboard
    C. After administration the remaining stock must be checked by a second person
    D. The total ward stock of this drug must never exceed 2 grams.

336.

337. 50 mg is equal to:
    A. 50000 micrograms
    B. 5000 micrograms
    C. 5 grams
    D. 0.5 gram.

337.

338. Before administering a dose of pethidine to Miss Maggs, which of the following is the most important duty of the nurse giving the drug?
    A. Inquire if the patient is in pain
    B. Inquire if the patient is nauseated
    C. Check when the last dose was given
    D. Check the last reading of the blood pressure.

338.

Miss Maggs made an extremely good recovery. Her niece visited her on the first postoperative day and said that she had arranged to stay on at the cottage and care for her aunt when she was discharged from hospital. Miss Maggs was very pleased with this news and even more pleased to know that Minnie was being well cared for.

339. Different surgeons vary in the time lapse before a patient is allowed out of bed after surgery, but the main principle is always the same. This is, to commence getting the patient out of bed:
   A. As soon as possible
   B. As soon as the danger of all postoperative complications has passed
   C. Directly she is capable of weight-bearing
   D. After she has completed a full course of physiotherapy.

339.

340. Before Miss Maggs left hospital, the medical social worker visited her again as Alice had wondered if her aunt could claim supplementary benefit. Apart from the cottage her only assets were £500 in savings. With regard to this, which of the following statements is true?
   A. People with savings in the bank are not entitled to supplementary benefit, regardless of the amount
   B. Miss Maggs could not qualify for supplementary benefit because she owned her cottage
   C. Owning a property does not automatically debar someone from supplementary benefit entitlement
   D. People over the age of 70 years automatically have supplementary benefit added to their retirement pension.

340.

Fractured femur answers and explanations (Questions 281–340)

281. **A**   Of the options given, the first action of the person finding Miss Maggs should be to cover her with his/her coat or jacket (a). While it is important not to overheat a person suffering from shock, it is also important to prevent the person from becoming cold. Ideally a coat or jacket placed underneath Miss Maggs would have afforded greater protection from the cold ground, but it may not have been possible to move her. The next priority would be to ascertain her identity (D). The order of (B) and (C) is not critical and would depend very much on the circumstances.

282. **D**   Of the options given, (D) must take priority. Such points as a possible head injury or respiratory distress should always be considered. Oral fluids (A) should not be given and attempting to move her (B) may cause further injury. Temporary splinting (C) is unlikely to be necessary as the ambulance staff will have an inflatable splint with them.

283. **B**   Shock is a state in which there is a diminished supply of circulating fluid. In an attempt to compensate for this the heart beats faster. Therefore the pulse will be rapid. The skin will feel cold and clammy due to diminished peripheral circulation (B).

284. **D**   As has been stated, shock is a state in which there is less fluid circulating. This may be caused by:
1. Injury or surgery, causing direct loss of body fluid by bleeding.
2. Emotion, causing an excess amount of fluid to be drawn into the tissues.

From this it can be seen that Miss Maggs's shock was caused by trauma (injury) and emotion (fear).

285. **C**   A splint (A) would provide support for the injured limb, and should not be removed initially. An analgesic (B) cannot be given until it has been prescribed by the doctor. In order to take Miss Maggs's blood pressure (D) it would be necessary to remove her top coat. Her other clothes should be removed at the same time to avoid unnecessary movement (C).

286. **A**   Miss Maggs is in pain and among strange people. Her greatest need is to feel that these people are kind and caring. Establishing eye contact is an effective way of providing reassurance. It is quite pointless saying, 'Don't worry, we will notify your niece' (B), or, 'We will take care of your pension' (C), if the nurse saying these words is looking in another direction while speaking.

287. **D** All of the points listed are likely to cause concern to Miss Maggs, but her greatest concern is likely to be for Minnie (the cat), as she will certainly need attention soon. We know from the introduction, that Miss Maggs considers Minnie's needs before her own (A and B), and while the garden may need attention at some time in the future, this will not be so urgent as Minnie's need for nourishment.

288. **D** It is a common belief that only people requiring an ambulance (A) are charged this fee, but this is not true. Every person involved in an accident with a licensed vehicle on the highway is liable to be charged the fee (D).

289. **C** Again, it is commonly believed that this fee is charged for the maintenance of ambulances (B), but this is not true. The Road Traffic Act states that this fee is to provide payment for the services of the first doctor attending the patient. It should be noted that the fee is small (less than £2 at the time of writing).

290. **B** Motor vehicles must be licensed and have road insurance, but bicycles need not.

    The answer for question 288, shows why (B) is the correct answer for this question.

291. **C** The terms 'fracture' and 'broken' both mean the same, and one does not indicate greater severity than the other (A, B and D). In practice lay people are more familiar with the term 'broken' which is why an elderly lady who has a fractured femur, may be told that she has broken her leg.

292. **C** The joint capsule surrounds the head and neck of the femur. Therefore
293. **B** fractures in this area are said to be intracapsular (within the capsule)
(292C). However this term does not indicate whether the head or neck
is fractured, so a more accurate way of describing Miss Maggs's injury
would be 'fractured neck of femur' (293B). Extracapsular fractures
(292D) are beyond the capsule and may be either intertrochanteric
(involving the trochanter (292A)) or subtrochanteric (below the
trochanter (292B)).

Intracapsular and extracapsular fractures
of the upper extremity of the femur

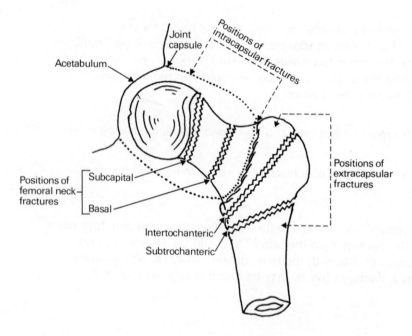

294. **B** Osteoporosis (loss of bone density (B)) is the most common
contributory cause. Paget's disease (thin, brittle bones, (C)) increases
the individual's susceptibility to fractures, but is a less common
condition. Osteomyelitis (inflammation of the bone (A)), and
Parkinsonism (a syndrome associated with the nervous system (D)) are
both less common conditions.

295. **D** Fractures of the neck of femur frequently result in a reduction of the
blood supply to the femoral head (D). This is because the main blood
supply comes from arteries which enter the femur at the junction of the
head and neck. Fractures may cause these blood vessels to become torn
and so disrupt the blood supply.

296. **B**   Miss Maggs is elderly, and in order to prevent complications due to prolonged bed rest, it is important that her treatment allows her to become mobile as soon as possible. In view of this, she is most likely to have an internal fixation of the fracture as soon as her general condition will allow it. She will certainly need physiotherapy and probably skin traction until she is fit for surgery (B). Skeletal traction (C and D) is more commonly used for fractures of the shaft of femur and plaster of Paris (A and C) for fractures of the tibia and fibula. Occupational therapy (C and D) is unlikely to be necessary in Miss Maggs's case.

297. **D**   A rigid mattress support (D) must be in position before Miss Maggs is put into bed, as it would cause her unnecessary pain and distress to be moved onto one later. A bed cradle (A) and bed blocks (B) could be added later without causing discomfort to the patient. A Balkan beam is not always required for patients with this type of fracture (C).

298. **C**   The best position in which to nurse Miss Maggs is semirecumbent. The prone position (B) would only cause distress and the left lateral (D) increase pain. The upright position (A), although it may help prevent pneumonia is not advocated for an elderly person with poor muscle tone. Miss Maggs would slip down very easily causing shearing forces which cut off the capillary network in the skin with resulting sores. The upright position is also contraindicated because she has recently been in a state of shock.

299. **B**   The semirecumbent position will help prevent the formation of sores due to friction (B). The rigid mattress and traction will help support the injured limb (D). Good physiotherapy will help prevent hydrostatic pneumonia (A) and some pain is inevitable (C).

300. **C**   Callus formation (A) and repair of periosteum (B) are of little concern if the patient is to have open surgery. But it is important that the patient's general condition is fit for surgery (C) (e.g. recovery from her state of shock).

301. **A**   Pugh traction is a simple form of balanced skin traction (A). Remember both skin and skeletal traction may be either 'fixed' (between two fixed points) or 'balanced' (sliding).

302. **D**   Skin traction may be applied by using either elastoplast or ventfoam extensions (C and D). As Miss Maggs is elderly, and the traction will only be used for a few hours, ventfoam (D) would be the best choice as this would reduce the risk of damaging her skin when the traction is removed. Steinmann pins and Denham pins are both used for skeletal traction (A and B).

303. **D** When a patient has a fractured femur, the leg is abducted (away from the mid-line) and laterally rotated (turning onto the lateral aspect (D)). Adduction means towards the mid-line, and internally rotated means turning onto the medial aspect.

Note: lateral—outer; medial—inner.

304. **C** When applying a bandage over ventfoam traction, all of the options are important, but the most important one is to ensure that the bandage is applied with even pressure (C) (not too tight or too loose). A bandage which is too tight may restrict the blood supply, and a bandage which is too loose will be ineffective.

305. **B** The reason for elevating the foot of the bed after applying traction is to apply countertraction (B) (the weight of the patient's body pulling in the opposite direction). If it had been necessary to elevate the foot of the bed to reduce the effects of shock (A) or oedema (D), this would have been done immediately. The most effective way of preventing the weights touching the floor (C) is to shorten the traction cords as they stretch!

306. **D** The medical social worker would need to assess the general situation (D) before any action could be taken (A, B and C).

307. **A** Rehabilitation means preparing a person to reach the maximum degree of physical and psychological independence of which she is capable. This programme of preparation should commence as soon as a person is admitted to hospital (A). For example, relief of pain can do much to restore a patient's confidence in her ability to recover.

308. **C** A private cats' home (A) could be very expensive, and the veterinary surgeon (B) would be unlikely to be able to accommodate Minnie as he cares for animals that are ill. Even the suggestion of having Minnie 'put to sleep' (D), would cause great distress to Miss Maggs and would probably cause a deterioration in her condition. From this it can be seen that the most appropriate action would be to ask the RSPCA for help (C). Frequently neighbours are able to help in situations like this, but we know that Miss Maggs's cottage is isolated.

309. **D** If a person is receiving DHSS retirement pension, it is necessary to notify the Department when she is admitted to hospital. However the pension is not likely to be reduced until the stay in hospital exceeds eight weeks (D). This rule applies to both general and psychiatric hospitals.

Note: different rules apply for supplementary pensions.

310. **C**   Nurses must always remember the importance of keeping all information about their patients in strict confidence. For this reason, it is usual for enquiries from the press to be referred to the hospital administrator. This does not mean that he is exempt from maintaining confidentiality, but simply that his training prepares him for dealing with this type of situation.

311. **D**   The law as to the witnessing of Wills requires that the signature of the Testator (the person making the Will) should be witnessed by two persons both of whom should be present together when the Testator signs it, and both of whom should sign as witnesses in the presence of the Testator. There is no legal requirement that the witnesses or either of them have to be solicitors, bank managers, priests or members of any other profession or occupation. A person who is a beneficiary under the Will should not sign it as a witness.

312. **C**   It is mainly to protect the nurse from being asked to testify in Court if a Will is contested, that hospital authorities discourage nursing staff from witnessing patients' Wills. If a patient asks to have a Will witnessed the hospital administrator will normally arrange for this.

313. **D**   All of the options listed are contributory factors to pressure sores forming, but the main cause is immobility (D). Remember, a thin, undernourished person may be active and not develop pressure sores, but the same person may develop a sore rapidly if confined to bed.

314. **D**   The most effective way of preventing pressure sores is to relieve pressure! Passive limb movement (A) will not relieve pressure from the sacral area. While use of the lateral (C) and prone (B) positions would be an effective method of relieving pressure for some patients, it would be inappropriate for Miss Maggs, because of her injury. By using her trapeze frequently (D), pressure would be relieved from the shoulders and heel as well as the sacral area.

315. **C**   Of the options listed, a full-length sheepskin (C) would be the most suitable for Miss Maggs, as this would relieve pressure from her sacrum, heels, shoulders and elbows. An air ring (D) would only be effective for her sacral area. A Stryker frame (B) is more suitable for patients with spinal injuries, and a water bed (A) would be unsuitable because of the need for traction.

316. **A**   The three main causes of pressure sores are pressure, moisture and friction. Having relieved pressure it is important also to keep the skin clean and dry (A). Spirit (B) should not be used as this dries the natural oils of the skin and causes it to crack. A good fluid intake (C) will help in keeping the skin supple, but will not prevent pressure sores if the skin is moist and dirty. While it is important to keep Miss Maggs free from pain, this may increase the risk of pressure sores, as she is less likely to move.

317. **B**   Miss Maggs would be most upset if she thought that the nurse was expecting her to 'make a mess' (D)! She would also be alarmed to be told that her leg was tied to the bed (A) and it is wrong to coerce a patient into doing something by making a promise that cannot be kept (C). Miss Maggs will be far more likely to co-operate if she is gently reminded why she cannot walk on her leg (B).

318. **C**   It is essential to reassure Miss Maggs and gain her co-operation, (C) because she will find it painful to be moved and will probably try to avoid being moved. To remove blankets from the bed (D) may cause the patient to become cold. Five centimetres from the mattress (B) is not high enough to lift a patient, and bedpans should never be 'pushed' into position, as the friction is liable to damage the patient's skin. If a cold bedpan is used (A), Miss Maggs will certainly feel it on her buttocks, even if her legs are protected by bandages.

319. **C**   It has just been said that a patient's skin can be damaged if a bedpan is pushed into position. The same thing can happen if a patient is left for too long on a hard bedpan or if a bedpan is positioned so that it comes into contact with a bony prominence. Once the skin has been damaged (either broken or bruised) a pressure sore may develop rapidly, because the skin in that area is deprived of vital nourishment to aid healing. Traction cords should not be released for simple nursing tasks (B) as this will delay union of the fracture and may also cause the patient unnecessary pain. There are many causes of urinary tract infection (A). Of these catheterisation is one of the more common causes.

It should be remembered that the risk of deep vein thrombosis is increased because Miss Maggs is unable to move her injured leg (D).

320. **D**   Providing the nurses are careful, Miss Maggs may be rolled onto either side (D). Care must be taken to support her body well, using the hands and arms. Once again, it must be remembered that Miss Maggs will need much reassurance as she will find it painful to be moved. Often the best plan is to allow the patient to choose which side she would prefer to rest on.

321. **D**   When a patient becomes restless in the night it may be due to any of a variety of reasons, e.g. pain, a full bladder, fear. Only by finding the cause of the patient's restlessness can the nurse take appropriate action (D). Neither sedation (C) nor cot sides (A) would be appropriate for the patient who wishes to empty her bladder.

322. **A**   Of the options given, a nail-plate would be used (A). The nail secures the fracture and the plate attaches the nail to the shaft of the bone giving greater stability. Intramedullary nail (C) is used for fractures of the femoral shaft, and a Steinmann pin (D) is used for securing skeletal traction. A prosthesis (B) may be used for replacing the femoral head following a fracture of the femoral neck but this is not the same as internal fixation of the fracture. (In the former the broken part of bone is removed, while in the latter it is secured in position.)

Fracture secured by nail plate

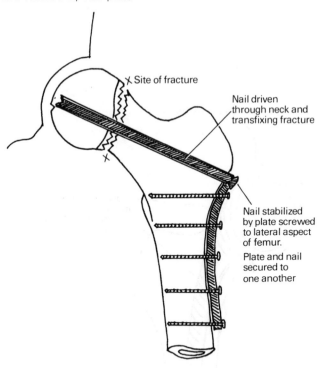

Internal fixation of fracture of the shaft of the femur

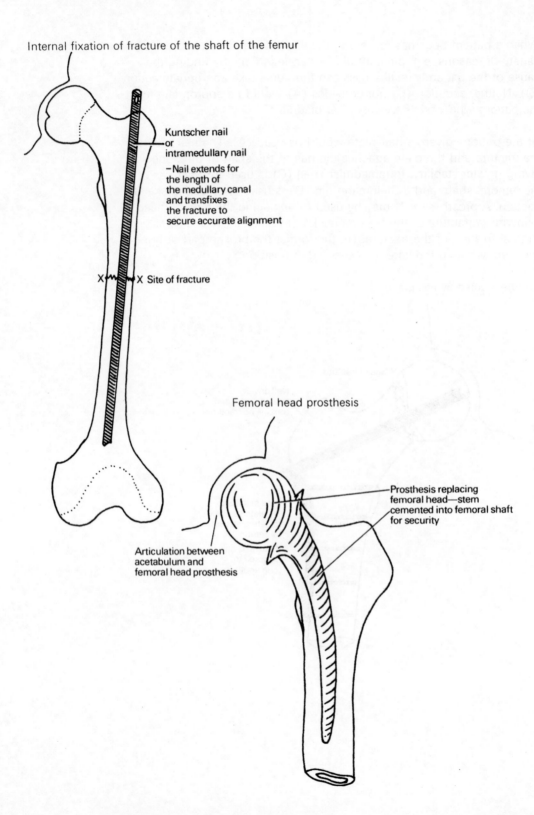

Kuntscher nail
or
intramedullary nail

−Nail extends for
the length of
the medullary canal
and transfixes
the fracture to
secure accurate alignment

X X Site of fracture

Femoral head prosthesis

Prosthesis replacing
femoral head—stem
cemented into femoral shaft
for security

Articulation between
acetabulum and
femoral head prosthesis

323. **A**   The first action of the nurse should be to check the patient's identiband. This is a safeguard against preparing the wrong patient for operation. From this it can be seen that it would be dangerous to give the premedication (B) or remove the traction (D) before correctly identifying the patient.

324. **B**   Normally we are able to control our bladder sphincter muscles. An anaesthetic renders the patient unconscious. An unconscious person loses control of the sphincter muscles which will then relax and the bladder will empty. A person who is incontinent of urine has lost normal bladder control.

325. **A**   It takes approximately three hours for a mixed meal to be digested in
326. **A**   the stomach. Therefore the minimum time for withholding oral fluids
327. **C**   would be four hours, as this would ensure that there is no food residue in the stomach. The reason it is important for the stomach to be empty is to prevent the possibility of vomiting during or immediately after the anaesthetic. The real danger of this is that the patient, being unconscious will be unable to eject the vomit from the mouth and may inhale it into the lungs.

328. **A**   If an event like this should happen, the priority is to ensure that the patient is not given an anaesthetic until appropriate action has been taken. Therefore the first action of the nurse in charge of the ward must be to notify the anaesthetist (A). You may argue that Sister is really in charge of the ward even if she is at lunch (B). Obviously she should be told what has happened as soon as possible, but if you telephone her first it may just happen that another nurse unknowingly takes Miss Maggs to theatre while you are speaking to Sister. To stay with Miss Maggs until Sister returns (D) would cause unnecessary delay.

329. **C**   There are 1000 micrograms to 1 milligram. To find the answer to the questions it is necessary to multiply 0.6 (milligrams) by 1000 (micrograms):

$$0.6 \times 1000 = 600.$$

330. **C**   Atropine has many effects including reducing spasm in plain muscle,
331. **C**   reducing salivary and bronchial secretions (330C), and dilating the pupil of the eye. The purpose of giving atropine as a premedication is to reduce bronchial secretions.

Because of its effect on the eye, it is important for the nurse preparing an injection of atropine to cover the tip of the needle while expelling air from the syringe (331C). Failure to do this may result in the nurse having difficulty with vision due to spray from the needle entering her eye.

332. **B**   This question deals with priorites. The identiband (C) and operation gown (D) should both have been dealt with before giving the premedication. Ideally after giving a premedication curtains should be drawn around the bed and the patient left to sleep (A), but there may be occasions when it is preferable not to completely close the curtains (e.g. a confused patient). However the nurse must always keep the patient under close observation (B), otherwise how is she to know if the drug is being effective or producing possible side effects?

333. **A**   This question is also dealing with priorities. All of the options listed are important for the care and well being of the patient, but the nurse must know what operation has been performed in order to plan care effectively. (Think of the stages of the nursing process.)

334. **C**   This question is also designed to establish priorities. All of the options listed must be attended to but the main point must be to ensure that the patient is in a fit condition for the journey (C). If problems occur, it may be that some of the points need checking more than once, but there must always be a final check on the patient's general condition (e.g. colour, rate and depth of respiration).

335. **C**   If the patient's jaw is held well forward the tongue cannot slip back. The same principle applies as in first aid, when it is necessary to extend the patient's neck to open the airway before giving mouth to mouth resuscitation. An artificial pharyngeal airway (A) is only effective if it is patent (e.g. not obstructed by blood or mucus). To administer oxygen (B) would be pointless until the obstruction of the airway has been removed. A cuffed endotracheal tube (D) is normally only used when a patient needs 'assisted respiration'.

336. **C**   Under the Misuse of Drugs Act 1971, pethidine is classed as a 'controlled drug'. In hospital, after administration of this drug the remaining stock must be checked and witnessed by a second person (C). Every nurse should be familiar with the Controlled Drugs Register used for this purpose. Drugs must not be allowed to accumulate in wards and care must be taken when ordering. The ward stock held of any particular drug will vary according to the needs of ward or department (D).

337. **A**   1 milligram is equal to 1000 micrograms. Therefore 50 milligrams is equal to 50000 micrograms (50 × 1000).

   Note: if you choose either (C) or (D) as your answer:
   1000 milligrams is equal to 1 gram.
   Therefore 5 grams is 100 times greater than the prescribed dose and 0.5 gram is 10 times greater than the prescribed dose.

338. **C**   As pethidine is an analgesic, it is important for the nurse to ask if the patient is in pain before administering a dose (A). However, her most important duty is to check when the last dose was given (C), otherwise there is a very real danger that the patient may receive an overdose, by being given two doses without sufficient time lapse between them.

339. **A**   The risk of some postoperative complications increases with the length of time a patient stays in bed (B), e.g. pneumonia, deep vein thrombosis. Some patients may not be able to bear weight on their injured leg (C) but this need not prevent them being lifted out of bed into a chair. Physiotherapy will be continued for some time after the patient is allowed out of bed (D), as it is important for the patient to regain a full range of movement. From this it can be seen that the main principle is to commence getting the patient out of bed as soon as possible (A).

340. **C**   Owning a property does not automatically debar someone from supplementary benefit entitlement (C). Many other factors are also taken into account; such as the person's annual income, including interest from certain savings (A). These factors need to be taken into account, regardless of the age of the person (D).

Rheumatoid arthritis

The following questions (341–387) are based on the case history given below:

Mrs Louisa Skinner was 43 years old when she first developed symptoms of arthritis. She lived with her husband in a third floor, rented flat. The flat was in an older style building with large, draughty rooms, high ceilings and a wide twisting staircase.

Mr Skinner was employed as a grower at a nearby small garden centre and Mrs Skinner had part-time employment, washing up in a local cafeteria. For the past three weeks, Mrs Skinner had been aware that the joints of her fingers were 'swollen and painful. In fact all her joints seemed to ache especially her wrists, knees and feet. On waking in the mornings her joints were so stiff that she felt unable to move, and more recently she had been feeling tired, depressed and generally unwell.

Mrs Skinner stayed at home from work for a few days but did not feel any better, so her husband persuaded her to visit the family practitioner who diagnosed rheumatoid arthritis.

Note. This case history covers a span of 11 years. However, the questions have been designed so that they should all be read as if the situation described was the present day.

Multiple choice questions

The following questions (341–387) are all of the multiple choice type. Read the questions and from the possible answers select the ONE which you think is correct. You may indicate your answer by writing the appropriate number in the space provided or against the question number on your answer sheet.

341. Which of the following statements is true?

    Rheumatoid arthritis is:
    A. Equally common in both sexes
    B. More common in women than men
    C. Rare in young adults
    D. Never occurs in children.

341.

342. Rheumatoid and osteoarthritis differ in that, 'rheumatoid arthritis':
    A. Is usually associated with systemic disturbance
    B. Usually results from injury to a joint
    C. Affects mainly larger weight bearing joints
    D. Is a progressive, non-inflammatory condition.

342.

343. Recent research indicates that arthritis may be an autoimmune disease.   343.
     Which of the following statements most accurately describes the process of
     autoimmunity?
     A. A rare complication of vaccination when the body reacts to the vaccine
        by producing symptoms of the disease
     B. An inherent factor in the blood which renders the person susceptible to
        certain diseases
     C. Lack of antitoxins in the blood which renders the person susceptible to
        certain diseases
     D. Formation of antibodies in the blood which destroy certain healthy cells
        of the individual

344. With reference to rheumatoid arthritis, which of the following statements is   344.
     true?
     A. There is no known cure for this condition
     B. A common complication of this condition is damage to the valves of the
        heart
     C. Primary symptoms occur within 10 days of the patient having a
        haemolytic streptococcal infection
     D. Involvement of the joints of the cervical vertebrae is rare.

345. Patients with rheumatoid arthritis commonly complain of stiffness of the   345.
     joints. With reference to this, which of the following statements is a typical
     history, as given by the patient?

     'The stiffness is':
     A. Better after resting
     B. Bad in the morning and gets worse as the day progresses
     C. At its worst in the morning and improves as the day progresses
     D. Present all the time and keeps me awake at night.'

The family practitioner gave Mrs Skinner a prescription for
analgesics and said that he would make an appointment for her to
attend the local rheumatology clinic as an outpatient. Mrs Skinner
asked if she could have transport provided to take her to the clinic
as she had found the journey by bus to the surgery today very
tiring. The doctor said he would arrange transport.

---

346. Which of the following analgesics is most commonly prescribed for patients   346.
     with rheumatoid arthritis?
     A. Aspirin
     B. Pethidine
     C. Arlef (flufenamic acid)
     D. Ponstan (mefanamic acid).

347. If the correct answer has been selected for question 346, which of the
following instructions should be given to the patient?
A. If dental treatment is required, tell the dentist about the drug being taken
B. Do not drive within four hours of taking the drug
C. Notify the doctor of any symptoms of dyspepsia
D. Rest on the bed for an hour immediately after taking the drug.

347.

348. With reference to payment for a National Health Service prescription, which
of the following statements is true?
A. Prescriptions are dispensed and issued free of charge
B. A nominal fee is charged for all prescriptions to cover the cost of bottles
and packaging
C. Children, expectant mothers and those drawing retirement pension or
supplementary benefit are all entitled to claim exemption from
prescription charges
D. Exemption from prescription charges is only permitted for those suffering
from a chronic illness or war disability.

348.

349. Provision of an ambulance service for transporting patients to the
outpatients clinic is the responsibility of the:
A. Social services department
B. Local government
C. Hospital management team
D. Area health authority.

349.

350. Drivers for the hospital car service are a team of:
A. Trainee ambulance staff
B. Retired ambulance staff
C. Social workers
D. Voluntary workers.

350.

351. With reference to payment for hospital transport to attend an outpatient
clinic, which of the following statements is true?
A. The service is provided free of charge
B. A nominal fee is charged for car transport only, to cover the cost of
petrol
C. A nominal fee is charged for both car and ambulance transport
D. Only people living within a three mile radius of the hospital are charged
a fee for the provision of transport.

351.

352. Bearing in mind what we know of Mrs Skinner, which of the following
forms of transport would be most suitable for the doctor to request for her?
A. Ambulance (stretcher)
B. Ambulance (sitting)
C. Hospital car service
D. Whichever vehicle is available.

352.

In due course Mrs Skinner attended the outpatient clinic and the consultant rheumatologist arranged for her name to be placed on the waiting list for admission to hospital. The purpose of the admission was for rest and further investigations.

While Mrs Skinner was attending the clinic specimens of her blood were taken and sent to the laboratory.

353. One of the tests conducted on Mrs Skinner's blood was for the rheumatoid factor. With reference to this test, which of the following statements is true?
   A. The presence of this factor in the blood, positively confirms a diagnosis of rheumatoid arthritis
   B. This factor may be present in the blood with a wide variety of diseases including bacterial endocarditis and liver disease
   C. This factor is normally present in the blood of all persons and a lowered level indicates a diagnosis of some form of rheumatoid disease
   D. This factor is normally present in the blood of all persons, and a raised level indicates a diagnosis of rheumatoid arthritis.

353.

354. Another test conducted on Mrs Skinner's blood was for ESR (erythrocyte sedimentation rate). Normal ESR for a woman is within the range of:
   A. 3–5 mm in 1 hour
   B. 3–5 mm in 2 hours
   C. 7–12 mm in 1 hour
   D. 7–12 mm in 2 hours.

354.

355. Patients with rheumatoid arthritis commonly have a raised ESR. This is because:
   A. Arthritis patients usually have a degree of anaemia
   B. The electrolyte balance of the blood is disturbed
   C. Inflammatory conditions cause an increase in the number of white cells in the blood
   D. The rheumatoid factor increases the viscosity (stickiness) of the cells.

355.

By the time Mrs Skinner was admitted to hospital, four months had passed since the onset of her symptoms. During this time she had not been attending her part-time employment and had been continuing to take her analgesics as prescribed.

On admission to hospital, the Consultant prescribed complete bed rest, and a course of myocrisin (sodium aurothiomalate).

356. Myocrisin is a form of:
   A. Steroid
   B. Gold salts
   C. Analgesic
   D. Cytotoxic agent.

356.

357. The normal route of administration for Myocrisin is by:
   A. Slow rectal infusion
   B. Slow intravenous infusion
   C. Hypodermic injection
   D. Deep intramuscular injection.

357.

358. Mrs Skinner's prescription sheet read, 'Myocrisin 50 mg once a week for 20 weeks'. Assuming all doses were given, at the end of 20 weeks she would have received a total dose of:
   A. 0.5 gram
   B. 1 gram
   C. 1.5 gram
   D. 2 grams

358.

359. When a drug is prescribed to be given once a week, which of the following is the *most* important duty of the nurse in charge of the ward?
   A. Ensure that it is given with the early morning drug round so that it is not forgotten
   B. Make one person responsible for ensuring that the drug is given regularly
   C. Ensure that the drug is given on the same day of each week (e.g. Sunday)
   D. Make certain that it is recorded in writing each time the drug has been given.

359.

360. Before each dose of Myocrisin is given, the nurse must inspect the
condition of the patient's skin because patients being treated with this drug
are particularly likely to develop:
A. Petechial patches
B. Pressure sores
C. Furuncles
D. Rashes.

360.

361. It is also important for patients being treated with Myocrisin to have their
urine tested regularly. With reference to this which of the following must
the nurse be especially careful to test for?
A. Sugar
B. Ketones
C. Protein
D. Bilirubin.

361.

362. Regular blood tests are another important feature in the care of patients
being treated with Myocrisin. This is because the drug frequently:
A. Depresses the function of the bone marrow
B. Destroys healthy, mature red blood cells
C. Enhances the production of white blood cells
D. Depresses the function of lymphoid tissue.

362.

363. Which of the following points is it most important to explain to Mrs Skinner
at the beginning of her course of treatment with Myocrisin?
A. It may take 10–20 weeks before any general improvement is shown
B. This drug usually produces extremely good results in arresting the course
of the disease
C. Side effects are rare
D. The treatment may be rather painful and unpleasant.

363.

Mrs Skinner was in hospital for six weeks. During this time her general condition improved considerably. When she was discharged from hospital arrangements were made for the community sister to give her her weekly dose of Myocrisin. Arrangements were also made for Mrs Skinner to attend regularly at the outpatient clinic and the physiotherapy department.

364. Which of the following is of prime importance in the care of the patient during an *acute* (active) phase of rheumatoid arthritis?
   A. Rest the body and the affected limbs
   B. Rest the body but give vigorous active exercises to the affected limbs
   C. Apply splints to the affected limbs
   D. Encourage the patient to walk about the ward and increase her range of activity each day.

   364.

365. During the *acute* phase of rheumatoid arthritis, the patient should be nursed in which of the following positions?
   A. Upright
   B. Recumbent
   C. Lateral
   D. A variety of different postures.

   365.

366. All of the following accessories may be used in the care of a patient with rheumatoid arthritis, but which one is likely to provide greatest comfort for the patient?
   A. Ripple mattress
   B. Trapeze (monkey pole)
   C. Sand bags
   D. Bed cradle

   366.

367. Which of the following must the nurse be especially careful not to give to a patient with rheumatoid arthritis?
   A. A pillow under the knees
   B. Pillows between the legs
   C. A blanket next to the body
   D. A nylon nightdress.

   367.

368. With reference to physiotherapy, which of the following is of prime importance during the early *acute* phase of rheumatoid arthritis?
   A. Breathing exercises
   B. Active exercises of the affected limbs
   C. Passive exercises of the unaffected limbs
   D. Hydrotherapy.

   368.

369. When Mrs Skinner attended the physiotherapy department as an outpatient, she was given local applications of heat. The main purpose of this form of treatment is to:
   A. Produce sufficient temporary relief of pain to enable the patient to perform her exercises
   B. Increase the range of movement of the affected joints without the need of active exercises
   C. Increase the supply of white cells to the affected joint and so reduce inflammation.
   D. Reduce swelling of the joint.

369.

Six years passed and brought many changes to Mrs Skinner's life. Her hands and feet were now very badly affected with arthritis, as were her knees and hips. Her increasing disability had made it necessary for the Skinners to be moved to a ground floor council flat, where several adaptations had been made to help her maintain a degree of independence.

Mr Skinner was still employed at the garden centre as he had another four years to work before reaching retirement age.

Twice in recent years Mrs Skinner had been admitted to hospital. The first time for an arthrodesis of the left knee and the second time for an arthroplasty of the right knee.

370 The purpose of an arthrodesis is to provide a joint which:
   A. Has a full range of movement
   B. Has a limited range of movement
   C. Is stable but not movable
   D. Is movable but not stable.

370.

371. With which of the following activities is Mrs Skinner most likely to need help as a result of having had an arthrodesis of the knee?
   A. Putting on her shoes
   B. Using the toilet
   C. Washing her legs
   D. Cutting her toe nails.

371.

372. Following arthrodesis of the knee, the most difficult action for a patient to perform is:
   A. Standing
   B. Walking
   C. Rising from a chair to the standing position
   D. Turning over in bed.

372.

373. Whenever possible, surgeons prefer to perform an arthroplasty of the knee rather than an arthrodesis. The main reason for this is because an arthroplasty:
   A. Provides a greater degree of mobility
   B. Is a smaller and less painful operation
   C. Is associated with less risk of postoperative complications
   D. Requires a shorter period of bed rest in the early postoperative stage.

373.

Another five years passed during which time Mrs Skinner (now aged 54 years) became progressively more disabled. However, she enjoyed the feeling of being in her own home, and now that her husband had retired he was able to give her more attention.

The family were receiving full support from the community services.

Mrs Skinner was still attending the outpatient combined clinic regularly and, on her last visit, it had been decided to arrange her urgent admission to hospital for surgery of the left hip.

In due course Mrs Skinner was admitted to hospital and after full preparation was taken to the operating theatre for total replacement of her left hip joint.

---

374. Total hip replacement is one form of:
   A. Arthrodesis
   B. Cup arthroplasty
   C. Prosthetic replacement of the femoral head
   D. Prosthetic replacement of femoral head and of acetabulum.

374.

375. Which of the following is the most important duty of the nurse caring for Mrs Skinner in the *immediate* postoperative period?
   A. Maintain a clear airway
   B. Record her pulse and blood pressure 1/2 hourly
   C. Prevent her from moving her legs
   D. Ensure that any instructions from the surgeon concerning application of traction are carried out at once.

375.

376. Mrs Skinner had a blood transfusion in progress. Her blood group was group A. This means that in an emergency she could receive blood from:
   A. Any other group
   B. Any group except B
   C. Group A only
   D. Group A and O only.

377. Twelve hours after operation Mrs Skinner started shivering and complaining of pain in her back. Her pulse was very rapid. In these circumstances which of the following should the nurse do first?
   A. Take her temperature
   B. Give her an extra blanket
   C. Send for medical aid
   D. Stop the blood transfusion.

378. With reference to question 377, the most probable explanation for Mrs Skinner's symptoms would be:
   A. Infection of the urinary tract
   B. Reaction to the anaesthetic
   C. An allergic reaction to the blood transfusion
   D. An allergic reaction to the metal prosthesis.

379. Mrs Skinner had wound drainage in position connected to a vacuum drainage bottle. With reference to this form of drainage, which of the following is the most important duty of the nurse?
   A. Ensure that there is a level of fluid at the bottom of the bottle at all times
   B. Ensure that the bottle is always well supported during nursing procedures
   C. Close the clip on the rubber tubing before lifting or turning the patient
   D. Keep the patient in the upright position to assist drainage.

380. A nurse notices that Mrs Skinner's wound drainage bottle has not accumulated any more fluid during the last two hours although it was functioning well before then. Which of the following should she do first?
   A. Check the position of the vacuum indicator (antenna) on the bottle
   B. Check the position of the metal (or plastic) clip on the bottle
   C. Inspect the patient's dressings for signs of seepage
   D. Move the patient to relieve any possible pressure on the drainage tube.

381. When changing a patient's vacuum wound drainage bottle, which of the following is the most important duty of the nurse?
   A. Maintain an aseptic technique throughout the procedure
   B. Ensure that the vacuum on the old bottle is exhausted before disconnecting it
   C. Clean around the rubber connection on the drainage tube with a suitable antiseptic
   D. Ensure that the old bottle is no more than three-quarters full of fluid.

Once Mrs Skinner had regained consciousness she was allowed to lie in bed without splintage or traction. A small firm pillow was placed between her malleoli.

382. The most probable purpose of placing a pillow between the malleoli was to:
    A. Prevent pressure sores
    B. Assist lateral rotation
    C. Maintain abduction
    D. Provide greater comfort.

382.

Mrs Skinner made a good postoperative recovery and was discharged from hospital four weeks after her operation.

For a while she made very good progress at home but then her condition started to deteriorate again. A year after her total hip replacement, the consultant prescribed oral prednisolone 5 mg daily for Mrs Skinner. This had a very good effect and she is still enjoying the independence of living in her own home, although she sometimes feels rather anxious about her future.

383. Prednisolone is a form of:
    A. Steroid
    B. Salicylate
    C. Diuretic
    D. Iron.

383.

384. Prednisolone is used in the treatment of rheumatoid arthritis if other methods have failed because its action is:
    A. Anti-inflammatory
    B. Antispasmodic
    C. Muscle relaxing
    D. Vasodilating.

384.

385. Special attention must always be paid to the safe keeping of drugs in the home. *Apart from the normal rules for safety,* which of the following is an additional necessity particularly relevant to the storage of prednisolone?

    The tablets should be:
    A. Kept in a glass container
    B. Stored in a refrigerator
    C. Stored in a warm place
    D. Protected from light.

385.

386. In the very early stages of treatment with prednisolone, patients commonly develop a state of:
    A. Depression
    B. Euphoria
    C. Anorexia
    D. Lethargy.

386.

387. Many aspects of her life would cause Mrs Skinner to be anxious about her future but which of the following is the most probable cause of greatest anxiety to her?
    A. The knowledge that other forms of treatment have brought about temporary relief, only to fail later.
    B. The knowledge that she is now totally dependent on the care given to her by her husband
    C. Fear of developing side effects to prednisolone
    D. Fear that she may need to have further surgery at a later date.

387.

Rheumatoid arthritis answers and explanations (Questions 341-387)

341. **B**   Rheumatoid arthritis is two or three times more common in women than in men. The average age of onset is about 40 years, although it can occur at any age. When children are affected by rheumatoid arthritis it is known as Still's disease.

342. **A**   Rheumatoid arthritis is a progressive inflammatory condition affecting the joints. Initially the small joints are affected but later the knees, hips, elbows and shoulders may be affected. Other systems of the body are affected by the inflammatory process, causing the patient to have various symptoms of systemic disturbance.

By contrast, osteoarthritis is a degenerative condition of larger weight-bearing joints and is not normally associated with systemic disturbance.

343. **D**   Normally the body is protected from infection by the immunity system. Organisms gaining entry to the body stimulate the lymphocytes to produce antibodies and antitoxins which destroy the invading organisms. Autoimmunity is a malfunctioning of this system, causing the immunity mechanism to produce antibodies against the body's own tissues.

344. **A**   Patients with rheumatoid arthritis commonly have periods of remission. Drugs do much to alleviate the symptoms but there is no known cure for the condition. As the disease progresses, joints of the cervical vertebrae (D) are frequently involved.

Primary symptoms of *rheumatic fever* occur within 10 days of the patient having a haemolytic streptococcal infection (C), and this condition is commonly complicated by damage to the valves of the heart (B).

345. **C**   If you have ever had a septic finger, you will know that the pain and swelling causes you to avoid using the finger, and this inactivity causes a feeling of stiffness. The principle is the same with joints affected by rheumatoid arthritis. When the person is asleep at night the joints are not being used, so that on waking there is an intense feeling of stiffness. As the day progresses, this stiffness gradually improves. Typically, by the end of the day the patient says the joints feel much better. She then goes to bed feeling more relaxed, and the whole process of inactivity causing stiffness starts again.

346. **A**   Despite the risk of side effects, aspirin (salicylic acid) is still the drug of
347. **C**   choice in the early stages of treatment for rheumatoid arthritis. This is
because its effects are anti-inflammatory as well as analgesic.

Arlef (346C) or Ponstan (346D) may be prescribed for arthritic pain,
but not as commonly as aspirin. Arlef is an anti-inflammatory drug and
Ponstan an analgesic but both are contraindicated in the presence of
gastrointestinal upset. Pethidine (346B) is a habit-forming drug and
would not normally be used for long-term treatment of arthritis. In order
to be effective, the aspirin needs to be given in large doses for a long
period of time, which increases the risk of side-effects—notably gastric
irritation, which may cause gastric ulceration and haemorrhage. For this
reason, it is very important for the patient to understand that she must
notify the doctor of any symptoms of dyspepsia.

348. **C**   Laws regarding payment for National Health Service prescriptions may
change with changing governments, but at the time of writing a
nominal charge is made for each item on a prescription. People in
certain categories may claim exemption from these charges. These
categories include children, expectant mothers, those drawing
retirement pension or supplementary benefit and also people suffering
from certain chronic illnesses (e.g. diabetes, epilepsy).

349. **D**   Provision of an ambulance transport system to take patients to and from
350. **D**   hospital is the responsibility of the area health authority. This applies
351. **A**   whether the patient is to be admitted to hospital, to attend an
outpatient clinic, or to attend one of the many hospital departments for
treatment. The ambulance crews are qualified staff, trained to lift and
move patients, and take appropriate action in an emergency. Drivers for
the hospital car service are a team of voluntary workers, who normally
use their own cars for this service. Although very able, willing people,
they should not be expected to lift or carry patients.

Hospital transport is provided free of charge regardless of whether it is a
car or ambulance, but can only be provided on the recommendation of
a doctor.

352. **B**   We know that Mrs Skinner lives in a third floor flat in an older style
building with a wide twisting staircase. If ambulance transport is
provided, an attendant will be available to help Mrs Skinner down the
staircase (A and B). We also know that Mrs Skinner is able to walk as
she attended the family practitioner's surgery, although she found it
tiring. From this it can be seen that a stretcher (A) would not be
required, as this would impose greater restrictions on her degree of
mobility.

Note: nurses are frequently asked to make decisions of this type when
ordering transport for patients to be taken home from hospital and it is
important to consider all the factors involved.

353. **B**   The rheumatoid factor is not normally present in the blood (C and D), but its presence does not positively confirm a diagnosis of rheumatoid arthritis (A). The factor may be present in the blood with a wide variety of diseases, including bacterial endocarditis and liver disease.

354. **C**   The test for estimating a patient's ESR is conducted by placing a
355. **D**   measured amount of blood in a test tube and allowing the cells to sink to the bottom. In women, the normal rate of sedimentation is 7–12 mm in 1 hour (in men, 3–5 mm in 1 hour). However, if the rheumatoid factor is present, it will cause the cells to be more 'sticky' so that they tend to cling together, the mass is heavier and so they fall more quickly.

356. **B**   Myocrisin is a form of gold salts. The normal route of administration is
357. **D**   by deep intramuscular injection.

358. **B**   To calculate the answer to this question, multiply weekly dose by number of weeks and divide by milligrams per gram.

There are 1000 milligrams in a gram.

$$\frac{50 \times 20}{1000} = \frac{1000}{1000} = 1 \text{ gram}$$

359. **D**   Any of the options listed may be used and quite frequently a combination of methods may be used, e.g. the drug is given with the early morning drug round (A) on the same day of each week (C). However, of the options listed the *most* important duty of the nurse in charge of the ward is to make sure that it is recorded in writing each time the drug is given. This not only ensures that the drug has been given, but also reduces the risk of the drug accidentally being given more than once a week.

360. **D**   Myocrisin is usually very effective in the treatment of rheumatoid
361. **C**   arthritis but unfortunately it is associated with a very high risk of serious
362. **A**   side-effects because it is excreted slowly. Many patients are unable to complete the course of treatment because they develop side effects and it is important for nurses to be aware of this when nursing a patient who is being treated with Myocrisin. Skin rashes are very common. In some cases renal failure may develop, which is why it is important to test the patient's urine regularly for protein. Myocrisin also depresses the function of the bone marrow so causing a deficiency of blood cells.

363. **A**   Myocrisin does not produce any immediate therapeutic effect and it may take several weeks of treatment before any general improvement is shown. It is important for the patient to understand this at the beginning of her course of treatment, otherwise she is likely to think that she is not responding to the treatment and this could make her very depressed.

364. **A** Rheumatoid arthritis is characterised by periods of acute activity of the disease and periods of remission. During the acute (active) stage of the disease other systems are involved and the patient is ill. During this stage, rest of the body and the affected limbs is of prime importance. There are varying opinions as to the amount of rest desirable as prolonged rest in bed may cause further complications. In some units it is the practice to enforce strict bed rest for three weeks, while others prefer regular rest periods during the day. During these periods, the patient will rest in bed with splints applied to the affected joints.

365. **D** The position of the patient will depend largely on which joints are most affected. A variety of positions should be used to prevent the common complications of pressure sores, joint contractures and chest infection. There is no 'hard and fast' rule that the patient should be nursed in any particular position, and the patient should be allowed to rest in whichever position she finds most comfortable, but correct body alignment should be maintained. The patient must not be allowed to lie with her knees bent up to her chest even if this is the most comfortable position.

366. **D** To answer this question, you need to think, 'what is making the patient *un*comfortable?'—stiff, swollen joints. The weight of bed clothes resting on these joints would make them even more painful. Using a bed cradle to take the weight of the bed clothes would relieve this, and therefore provide greatest comfort for the patient.

367. **A** Patients with arthritis frequently have a sensitive skin, due to the drugs they are taking (e.g. steroids) and for this reason many of them prefer not to wear a nylon nightdress (D), or have a blanket next to the body (C). Pillows between the legs (B) are commonly used when the patient is in the lateral position to prevent pressure. However, a pillow should not be placed under the knees of *any* patient, as this increases the risk of deep vein thrombosis. In patients with rheumatoid arthritis a pillow would increase the risk of flexion contractures of the knees.

368. **A** It has been stated earlier that during the acute (active) phase of rheumatoid arthritis rest is of prime importance. Prolonged rest in bed increases the risk of pneumonia and for this reason, breathing exercises are a very important part of physiotherapy. *Active* exercises (those the patient can do herself) would not be encouraged for the affected limbs (B); and *passive* exercises (gentle moving by the physiotherapist) would not be necessary for the unaffected limbs (C), as the patient could move these herself. Hydrotherapy (D) may be used at a later stage of treatment (e.g. after the acute phase).

369. **A**   Heat has no remedial property, but it does bring temporary relief of pain. For this reason heat is often applied to a very painful rheumatic joint in order to relieve pain and enable the patient to perform her exercises more effectively.

370. **C**   When a joint is fused (made immovable) it is called an arthrodesis.
371. **D**   From this it can be seen that Mrs Skinner would have had a knee joint
372. **C**   which was stable but not movable. Because she was unable to bend her knee, she would have found it extremely difficult to cut her toe nails. The other options in question 371 may have proved a little difficult, but there are many 'aids to daily living' available now, including raised toilet seats and long-handled shoe lifts.

Rising from a chair to the standing position is a very difficult action to perform following an arthrodesis of the knee joint (try sitting down yourself while keeping your knee in full extension, and then rising to the standing position without flexing the knee!).

373. **A**   When a patient is provided with a false joint, which is still movable, it is known as an arthroplasty. Surgeons prefer to perform this operation rather than an arthrodesis, whenever possible, because it allows the patient a greater degree of mobility.

374. **D**   It has already been said that an arthrodesis (A) is an operation fusing a joint, while an arthroplasty is an operation providing a false but movable joint. Arthroplasties of the hip may take the form of:

1. Replacing the acetabulum (B)
2. Replacing the femoral head (C)
3. Replacing both the acetabulum and the femoral head (D).

375. **A**   When caring for Mrs Skinner it is important for the nurse to record her pulse and blood pressure regularly (B); prevent her from moving her legs (C); and ensure that the instructions of the surgeon are carried out (D). But the *most* important duty of the nurse is to maintain a clear airway, as failure to do this could result in the patient's death.

376. **D**   The ABO system of blood grouping is determined by the presence or absence of two particular substances in the patient's red blood cells.

If one substance is present the blood is called group A.

If the other substance is present the blood is called group B.

If both substances are present the blood is called group AB.

If neither substance is present the blood is called group O.

A person with group AB blood is known as a universal recipient. She may safely receive blood from any of the other three groups but her blood must *never* be given to anyone who does not belong to the same group.

A person with group O blood is called a universal donor. She may safely give blood to anyone belonging to any of the other three groups but she must *never* receive blood which is not Group O.

Note: before a blood transfusion is given to a patient the rhesus factor must also be checked.

377. **D**   When a patient receives a transfusion of blood that is incompatible with
378. **C**   her own, an allergic reaction takes place and the blood cells clump together. This will make the patient very ill and may even cause death. The patient may have a high temperature, rapid pulse, jaundice and pain in the back. At the first indication of these symptoms the nurse should stop the blood transfusion and seek help immediately.

379. **B**   Whenever a wound drain is connected to a vacuum drainage bottle, it is important to ensure that the bottle is well supported during nursing procedures, otherwise the weight of the bottle will pull the tube and cause discomfort to the patient (normally a stitch is used to hold the drain in position). Keeping the patient in the upright position (D) is preferable when possible, but not essential. For this type of wound drainage it is not necessary to close the clip before moving the patient (C) or maintain a level of fluid at the bottom of the bottle (A).

380. **A**   Vacuum drainage bottles may be made of either glass or plastic. Whichever type is used, there is a small protruding indicator (antenna) at the top to show whether or not the vacuum is still present. If fluid is not accumulating in the bottle the nurse should check the position of this indicator (C). If the vacuum is still present she may then go on to check the other options listed.

381. **A**   The vacuum drainage bottle is connected to a tube which leads directly into the patient's wound. It is therefore essential for the nurse to maintain an aseptic technique when changing the bottle.

382. **C**   By placing a pillow or wedge between the malleoli the legs are held apart (abducted). This is an important feature in the postoperative care of a patient who has had a total hip replacement.

Note: lateral rotation (B) is *not* desirable, as this would increase the risk of dislocation.

383. **A**   Prednisolone is a form of steroid and has an anti-inflammatory action. It
384. **A**   is now rarely used in the treatment of rheumatoid arthritis, unless all
385. **D**   other forms of treatment have failed, because it carries a very high risk
386. **B**   of serious side-effects. When prednisolone is used it often brings about a dramatic improvement in the patient's condition. It is quite common for patients being treated with this drug to become euphoric (have an unrealistic sense of 'well being'). When storing prednisolone it is important to remember that it should be protected from light.

387. **B**   This case history has frequently illustrated the fact that Mrs Skinner enjoys being in her home and maintaining as much independence as she is capable of. She knows that she is only able to enjoy this, thanks to the devoted care of her husband. It is only natural that she should feel concerned for his well being, knowing that she is causing him a lot of extra work. When a person knows that they are totally dependent on the care given to them by a relative, it is not surprising that the person often has fears of what would happen to them if the relative was to be ill or die.